THE WAY OF

THE SKEPTICAL

NUTRITIONIST

OTHER BOOKS BY MICHAEL A. WEINER:

Earth Medicine—Earth Food

Plant a Tree

Man's Useful Plants

Nutritional Ethnomedicine in Fiji

Weiner's Herbal

The People's Herbal

Homeopathic Medicine

# *The* WAY OF THE SKEPTICAL NUTRITIONIST

A STRATEGY FOR DESIGNING YOUR OWN NUTRITIONAL PROFILE

MICHAEL A. WEINER

MACMILLAN PUBLISHING CO., INC.   NEW YORK

COLLIER MACMILLAN PUBLISHERS   LONDON

Macmillan Publishing Co., Inc.
866 Third Avenue, New York, N.Y. 10022
Collier Macmillan Canada, Ltd.

Library of Congress Cataloging in Publication Data
Weiner, Michael A.
    The way of the skeptical nutritionist.
    Bibliography: p.
    Includes index.
    1. Nutrition.   2. Diet.   I. Title.
TX353.W35   1981      613.2      81–2792
ISBN   0–02–625620–7          AACR2

10 9 8 7 6 5 4 3 2 1

Designed by Jack Meserole

Printed in the United States of America

For Janet, whose patience during these years
of my dietary turmoil far exceeded my own.
And, of course, for Russell and Rebecca,
who listened to the debates.

# CONTENTS

ACKNOWLEDGMENTS    ix

1    INTRODUCTION: WHY I AM A SKEPTIC    3

2    HEALTH AND DIET IN CONTEMPORARY
     PRIMITIVE POPULATIONS    13

3    THE ETHNIC FACTOR    18

4    ETHNIC DIETS FROM THE DISTANT PAST    36

5    OVERCOMING THE FAMINE WITHIN    49

6    WATER: THE UNIVERSAL NUTRIENT    105

7    ROOTS OF HEAVEN: ALCOHOL AND
     NUTRITION    113

8    FLIES IN THE SLAUGHTERHOUSE    124

9    KOSHER FOOD LAWS: TOWARD A REVISED
     INTERPRETATION    135

10   FOOD AS MEDICINE    141

11   DIET AND CANCER    177

*Book One*

NIGHT
DARKNESS

*Book Two*

DAWN
LIGHT

*Book Three*

MORNING
BRIGHTNESS

*Book Four* 12    AT THE NUTRITIONIST'S    199

NOON
CLARITY    13    A STRATEGY FOR DAILY DINING    215

14    "THE DIETARY DEBATE OF THE CENTURY":
ATKINS VS. PRITIKIN    225

15    HOLISTIC HEALTH: A HAVEN IN DEMISE?    229


POSTSCRIPT: ABOARD A SHIP TO
PANAMA    236


BIBLIOGRAPHY    238


INDEX    243

# ACKNOWLEDGMENTS

This excursion away from authoritarianism in nutrition owes its inspiration to my teacher, Dr. Sheldon Margen, who is not responsible for his student's theories and conclusions. Also, as always, Kathleen Goss has clarified my intent.

# Book One
## NIGHT DARKNESS

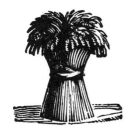

This book is likened to a heap of nuts. No sooner do you touch one, than all the rest start rolling. Likewise, when we attempt to answer some point of interest, we are overwhelmed with *all* questions of diet, nutrition, and health.

There is no scientific work that only one man can write.
—GALILEO

The ability to measure the heavens is won by doubt.
—GALILEO

# 1 INTRODUCTION: WHY I AM A SKEPTIC

Food is such a personal thing, and how anybody can dare suggest diets for others continually shocks me! And repugnant cuisine is scarcely the road to health and long life.

Now, there are fine books on becoming vegetarian. Some of my closest friends are vegetarians, yet we must *not* seek to declare as an objective truth that the plant world holds our major key to longevity. It may be true that George Bernard Shaw, Tolstoy, Wagner, Shelley, Byron, Thoreau, and other illustrious figures were vegetable eaters, but so was Hitler. In fact, the German dictator's manic-depressive mood swings and associated unexpected aggressive outbreaks might easily have been somewhat controlled with a good dose of high-quality protein and unrefined carbohydrates, and with a steady intake of a good vitamin/mineral supplement, on a regular basis. Better, he should have gnawed on a big leg of lamb once a day and had a glass of wine.

The well-known photo of Hitler and Eva Braun at Berchtesgaden, with the maniac passed out in an armchair after eating lunch, is *not* an image the hypoglycemically attuned researcher is likely to forget! Diet and behavior vary in too many people for us to look for a simple set of rules as our salvation from too intense swings of mood. Yet for a precious few types, as described later on, there *are* firm principles that can make the daily voyage much less erratic.

Nutritionists and others just now seeing the fortune to be made by pretending to *know* what you and I should eat—these honest practitioners of the physical arts would like us to believe that an objective set of rules, eternal truths even, exists regard-

3

ing diet and health, which, were we to follow, we would all live to the age of Moses.

Yes, there *are* patterns of disease related to certain foods and diets, and these are described, but we must proceed with some restraint lest we eliminate what is particularly required by our own peculiar idiosyncrasies of need. Those dietary totalitarians who would have us follow *their* branch of nutrition must be reminded that animals fed a "balanced" diet of all known nutrients will sicken and die while those allowed to forage live out their allotted spans. We vary enormously in our *specific* nutritional needs and must be allowed to follow our own dietary intuition once it has been somewhat reeducated.

Being one of the few doctors of nutrition, I must apologize for being too well versed in what is unknown to declare our shards of knowledge a firm mosaic of medical truth. I not only read scientific papers for truths, but also read people at first hand: in restaurants, at tables in homes, in hospitals, jails, crazy houses, trains, planes, and cafeterias. An unconventional way of studying diet and health, but a more complete method.

Some of my sources are my wife's great-grandfather, now ninety-six years old, who swims weekly, existing on a few, simple packaged foods; a Fijian agricultural worker, aged sixty, with the musculature of a twenty-year-old, who eats simple, unrefined foods of the islands; an old stranger in my favorite Chinese restaurant, whose lyrical neck and gait are reflected in his choice of steaming delicacies; a bear of an Italian woman who serves me in her North Beach restaurant, suggesting lamb chops for my digestion when I am not feeling too good; a deck steward I once met on a crossing between Honolulu and Vancouver; my now-deceased favorite uncle who dined primarily on vegetables; a New York heroin addict I grew up with who violates most health rules, but manages to play a fast game of tennis; most botanists, who seem to outlive nutritionists by at least twenty years; all primitive peoples; and any health teacher who does not kill our sense of curiosity in life or who has not killed it in herself or himself. . . .   I cannot enumerate them all.

The recent scandalous financial associations between some members of our "prestigious" National Academy of Sciences Food and Nutrition Board and various producers of cholesterol-rich foods (notably eggs and beef), and the attendant shift in recommendations about eating fats, reinforces my independent stance.

Courage is a rare virtue in a modern scientist. But I have always wandered between subjects, seeking to intertwine the frog and the tree, the religionist and the harlot, our demons and angels, and that gives me courage.

This is not to say that I am unimpressed with the "hard facts" of science. It is just a question of how "hard" and whose eye is doing the interpreting. Eight or more cups of strong, black coffee may drive most Westerners over the brink of nervousness, even bringing near-madness to the low-blood-sugar type, but this amount is considered moderate by my Bedouin Arab hosts in Israel. Those of us who sit and drive a lot may increase our heart-attack profile by eating vitamin $B_6$–deficient diets, while Eskimos and African milk-and-blood-eaters do quite well on fats, with scarcely a green leaf.

## A Cautionary Skepticism

In cajoling you to trust your instincts when it comes to what you should eat, a cautionary skepticism must be attached as a "rider." Our instinctual understanding of what is "good" for us has been somewhat garbled—by the forces of religion, culture, family, economics, and the influence peddlers; i.e., by "society." People generally follow stereotypical rules in their daily diet, such as: "When hungry, eat"; "What you strongly desire, does no harm"; "When the stomach calls, everything tastes good"; "If it tastes good, eat it"; "Avoid red meat, milk, and dairy"; and so on. Many of us have been conditioned to believe that everyone should follow his own tastes and inclinations and should loyally adhere to personal likes and to those habits formed in the early years.

But these habits are due to circumstances, or influences—good and evil—that have surrounded us since birth. Prevailing fashions in diet, local customs, current "scientific" notions, and our individual caprices and prejudices are all calculated to create artificial wants that often entail health-threatening and dangerous symptoms. How many of us, usually big meat-eaters, experience a sense of ungratified appetite, as though something were still wanting, when we have not gotten our favorite food to *excess?*

This dietary illusion is akin to those addicted to cocaine, heroin, alcohol, and nicotine. It is an illusion into which are apt to fall otherwise content folks who think that they are doing the right thing when, with a hearty appetite and a rich meal, they appease a merely imaginary craving that overloads their digestive and circulatory systems. The same mistake is made by the hard or stressed worker who drinks for the avowed purpose of bracing up for the job or presentation, or to compensate for a lack of food, but who no longer simply drinks for the sake of the pleasure and mild euphoria that follow.

Yet there must be certain laws, rules, or regulations by which we are to govern our diet. The food question is paramount in our life; our very existence is dependent upon it!

## Food Fascism

The bookstores are lined with "correct diets" for the unmet masses. Social engineers, having arranged our personal lives from sexual behavior to dying, have been aided in applying their golden rules to our last frontier: food. Food fascism, like other varieties of this social disease, requires lieutenants to proselytize. Not wishing to participate in any form of totalitarianism, I intend *not* to dictate a "correct diet" for a fictional reader!

This makes as good sense nutritionally as it does politically: for food needs are extremely individual once we learn to separate our *true* or biological food needs from what we have learned they are. Yes, there are general rules, both for the healthy and the sick, for the somewhat sick and the convalescent. Specifics are given for various disease states, but, for the healthy— well aside from a few general guidelines, a few shifts in relative *proportions* of desired foods, the inclusion of some protective foods, and minor supplementation—people should be left alone to exercise their last allowable freedom. Why? Because some of us are not as dumb as the doctors and nutritionists would have us believe! Dietitians are generally hopeless when it comes to devising adequate diets, as our hospital malnutrition will demonstrate. Anyone who uses a calculator to cook would be swiftly ushered from the kitchen of my hospital, let alone restaurant! Our tastes may be somewhat conditioned, and this we can overcome; they may be somewhat jaded, and this we can restore; but to reject with totality our wisdom for life is an utter absurdity, even in the shadow of nuclear totalitarianism.

## In Praise of Instinct

Instead of performing a rote set of neck and spine exercises, I choose to turn my head at every passing woman with the slightest charm! My neck and the egos of charming strangers are thus benefited by following this instinctual urge. Women rest in the palace of female tranquility, while I amble along impressed by my still too cavalier attitude.

Unfortunately, what works in the spinal department does not apply to diet. If I were to eat whatever "appealed" to me, on a daily basis, I would again suffer from the torturous migraines and insomnia induced by sucrose, a lock-and-key puzzle that took me four years to solve. Fat tastes good, but is so replete with cancer-causing substances (ingested by the animal, and formed during cooking) that I would surely risk my health by satisfying this craving. Elegant little French dishes satisfy only my need for entertainment. To properly follow our "instincts," we must learn how we have been influenced and then decide how to reprogram our tastes.

# Fabricated Foods: A Twentieth-Century Fantasy

We are cajoled into accepting fabricated foods not so much by forces that tend to have us *forget* the past as by forces that *distort* the past. Televised images of homey grandparents on their little bright farms gorging themselves on pies and hams, as well as frozen dinners, are a *distortion* of actual American farm meals, even in this country. Pies and hams were reserved for occasional meals, usually celebrations, and were not eaten as everyday foods.

But our acceptance of fabricated foods such as sawdust bread (an ITT contribution to man's health), imitation eggs, dehydrated infant formulas, synthetic meats, computerized beer and juice drinks, additive-rich wine, and so on, *is* a reflection of our desire not only to forget the past but to leap from the zoological order in which we were all born. We comply with these images because we wish to forget we are not angels, able to do just as we wish without penalty. And so the little that remains of our cultural ties is cast to the winds. By complying with media messages, the majority learns little and cares less about ancestral, even recent familial, menus. Instead of a disciplined attitude toward food, we rush to vitamins and special diet guides for our salvation. Yet only by looking to the past can we find our future roads.

## The Ethnic Factor

The current drift of nutritional thinking is an extension of the mechanistic world in which we live. By proposing a biochemical analysis of our blood, urine, and hair for vitamin, mineral, and blood-sugar content, current therapists then "prescribe" what is missing. Vitamin shots are given, multivitamins, minerals, hormones, and amino acids are prescribed on a maintenance schedule, and diets that are drastically removed from our senses are ordered to be followed to the end of time.

Whatever the biochemical wisdom of this approach—and there may *be* ultimate sense to megavitamins and related nutritional programs—we must remember that eating must also remain the great pleasure it is. Without our sense of smell alerting us to delicate flavors, the taste buds each delimiting the special characteristics of our next mouthful of pleasure, eating would soon become just one more task to accomplish in our already mechanical lives.

Food carries more than nutrients. Entire cultures are represented by characteristic foods. In addition to evoking images and sensations of cultural relationships, our food must also carry our personal histories as well. The psychological advantages lost when we remake our eating patterns may *not* be compensated for by the small biochemical pluses.

Woe to us if the biochemists devise a pellet containing all known and all suspected required nutrients! Then eating would be viewed as excessive indulgence, an unpatriotic, undemocratic greed in a malnourished world. What would we become but perfectly trim, absolutely healthy automatons with timetables for our every act, including death?

## How This Book Works

By the time you finish reading this book, you may know more than your doctor about nutrition.

Before you invest in a visit to a nutritionist, doctor, chiropractor, or other health consultant offering services in nutritional guidance, you must know how to evaluate the services being offered and, later, what to look for in your consultations.

Beginning with a look at what primitive people eat and the diseases they suffer from, the reader is taken on an odyssey through time, showing that man was not created to eat a highly specialized diet. We are made of strong, highly adaptable stuff and are able to live, even thrive, on a tremendous variety of foods. These notions that we are supposed to be vegetarians, or live without alcohol, are mere speculation, not supported by the evidence of archaeology. Worse are the proponents leading us to the trough of chemical food supplements, who would have us abandon eating itself, simply because we derive pleasure from the act.

We will come to see how our "ethnic factors" can be used to carry us to the proper diet. After a decade of research and travels I have concluded that ethnic diets have their own wisdom which belies the biochemical thrust of contemporary therapy. The science of nutrition may be likened to psychology when Freud first took his medical degree. Because nutrition is a field in its infancy, we are seeing many unproven theories of diet being offered as the ultimate, when the past may hold more direction regarding what to eat than will the future, where technicians and practitioners interested in selling supplements will lead us to believe that vitamin/mineral/amino-acid pellets can substitute for food as nutrition and emotional offering.

Have you ever wondered how prescription drugs interfere with specific nutrients? Or which nutrients you need if you continue to smoke? Would you like to see the kinds of home tap-water filters that are available? Have you decided if too much bran can interfere with calcium, iron, and zinc absorption? What about the RDAs? Do you really understand them, and how to interpret them on food packages? Are you a confirmed vegetarian, or macrobiotic? Do you keep kosher because you think it is better for your physical health? These essential questions are treated with crystal clarity in "Overcoming the Famine Within," a chapter essential in an age of dietary messiahs, each with her own platform.

The reader is guided not merely by theories, but by the author's observations and conclusions, based upon working with clients as a nutritional consultant, and upon visits with primitive peoples in the South Seas over a ten-year period.

Did you ever wonder why moderate drinkers outlive abstainers, *and* indulgers? Or which wines are particulary recommended for *your* nutritional profile? How about the additives in wine; would you like to know what they are, and what allergies they may be inciting? In the chapter, "Roots of Heaven," you will journey from the time of the accidental discovery of beer through the modern distilleries and decide which type of alcoholic beverage is the most beneficial instead of the least harmful.

In the old days "Flies in the Slaughterhouse" were the greatest threat to our food supply. In the chemical age, however, otherwise immaculate food-processing plants and restaurants are shown to be veritable storehouses of filth. You will learn how to avoid a sea of toxins without drastically changing your eating *patterns,* all the while reminded through delightful anecdotes set in restaurants, trains, planes, ships, straw huts, prisons, hospitals, and so on, that food can be a great pleasure, and must never become just a chore.

We all get sick on occasion, even the hardiest of us, and when we do, "Food as Medicine" may be our best choice, depending on the severity of our symptoms. Since physicians are often completely untrained in nutritional medicine, you will learn how to feed yourself and your family to avoid and treat various disease states. Topics discussed in this section include the hospital diet, diet and cancer, food allergies, diet and depression, impotence and diets, fasting, and orthomolecular medicine.

Having toured the state of the art in nutrition, you will be able to calculate your own nutritional needs, in Book Four. An interesting computerized dietary analysis of the foods you regularly eat will be explained in detail. You will learn the meaning of protein, fat, and carbohydrate in your diet, and how to modify your relative proportions to better balance your meals. Foods that are rich in the vitamins and minerals you may be lacking are also detailed, as is an analysis of your own caloric intake. You will be shown the various types of hair analyses utilized, and then be able to interpret intelligently the results of this technique; blood tests for nutrient levels are also described, as are some of the newer techniques you may encounter in your visit to a nutritionist. "A Strategy for Daily Dining," which is an intriguing condensation of the world's nutritional wisdom, is presented for your enjoyment and nutritional decision-making. This is followed by a critique of dietary messiahs, those would-be leaders who prove that their opposing positions are equally invalid, as are their dietary extremes.

In the final chapter an evaluation of dangerous trends in alternative medicine is offered in "Holistic Health: A Haven in Demise?" This should give you the ability to question with skepticism the theories, approaches, and advice of contemporary "healers," in an attempt to derive the greatest health benefits at the lowest cost and risk.

# The Magic and Mystery of Diet and Health: A Note to Scientists and Physicians

The mystery of life cannot be pressed into a pill or condensed in a book. No living thing was ever created by man, though surely life can be supported, or destroyed, by our actions and ingestions. What we eat will by no means save us when our time has come, but to keep that time from arriving is the entire purpose of wisdom in food and drink, or the abstention therefrom.

My idea is that ethnic diets were developed through the course of social evolution and have wisely adaptive health value. Food technologists and allied industrial forces are moving to obliterate our remembrance of these ethnic dishes in an attempt to standardize our food just as other totalitarian forces want to standardize man's behavior. *Control* is the key word. By standardizing food choices and then foods, a control is gained at loss of liberty. But worse, our health suffers. Looking at the degree of degenerative disease in the industrialized ("standardized") countries, I surmise that heart attacks, cancer, diabetes, alcoholism, some mental disease, and other major killers have vastly increased owing to the stress of conformity, in behavior and foods. Bypassing the wisely adaptive ethnic foods and patterns of the past, many of us have adopted a wholly unnatural rhythm, and eat foods for which *our* particular genetic makeup may be widely maladapted.

To "prove" this point, going against the current fad of biochemical explanations and concoctions, I rely on an impressionistic approach to the scientific facts that are based on firm experimental evidence. That is, my "proof" is just as firm, or just as questionable, as any other current notions about diet and health, when appraised on a strictly logical basis. The particular strength of my hypotheses comes from one major pillar, nearly always overlooked by other scientists: the irrefutable record of the past. I do not begin my discourse at some arbitrary period in our history as a species, but attempt to dig at the most ancient bones to arrive at the truth. Another of my particular strengths comes from my intensive study of man in all his diverse cultural forms. My earlier work as ethnobiologist strengthens my belief in the wisdom that many cultures have devised and carried through the ages. These adaptive strokes of genius, which center on various food combinations and avoidances, must not be thrown away in a single generation, lest we see the spread of civilization's worse diseases. Finally, strictly *intuitive* forces within me further fuel my argument that we, as a species, are adapted to many different diets and we weaken ourselves when we adopt strange dietary regimens for any length of time. My travels among many different peoples, and my nearly continual observation of how and what people eat, strengthen my desire to disavow the totalitarian strains now running through the medico-nutrition field.

# 2 HEALTH AND DIET IN CONTEMPORARY PRIMITIVE POPULATIONS

In the Kalahari, atop New Guinea mountains, across vast Australian deserts, on the slopes of the Andes, in the Philippine rain forests, and in other more limited geographies, populations exist with styles of living similar to those of prehistoric man. While many features of agricultural life have been adopted by these peoples, they are still sufficiently similar to our distant ancestors in their day-to-day living to warrant our interest.

Archaeological evidence and recent studies of aboriginal peoples indicate that the hunters and gatherers were the original leisure society, their food requirements being met by three or four hours of work a day. Studies of contemporary collecting peoples reveal that their diet is extremely varied. When they adopt agricultural practices, their diets become more simplified, generally centering around a starchy staple; since they must now attend to their crops and livestock, they lack the time for gathering wild foods. *Hunting and Gathering Efficient*

The recently discovered Tasaday of the Philippines are a good example of a hunting and collecting society. Before their contact with outsiders they subsisted on wild fruits and other plants, with animal protein coming from the fish, crabs, and frogs of the stream along which they lived, and palm grubs providing a good source of fat. Three or four hours of leisurely collecting a day, traveling no more than a kilometer from their cave homes, are sufficient to satisfy their dietary needs. The rest of their time is devoted to leisure activities. The Tasaday follow no fixed schedule for meals, snacking lightly throughout the day as they move about. Food is shared among the entire group as needed. This eating pattern seems to be ideally suited *Much Leisure Enjoyed by Tasaday* to the human digestive tract, which is able to operate more efficiently with frequent snacks than with heavy meals. Obesity is not a problem for the Tasaday, nor do they have a problem with tooth decay. The only diet-related disorder they appear to have is goiter; there are no other signs of nutritional deficiencies.

*Bushmen Adapt Well to Dietary Changes*

Other primitive peoples live in less fortunate environments, but still manage to subsist on the food they hunt and collect. Robson (1977), in a review of the available literature on this subject, observes that the Bushmen of the Kalahari experience seasonal fluctuations in their food supply, with the staple food being the high-protein and high-calorie mongongo nut. Comprising some eighty-five plant foods and some fifty-four different animal foods, the diet of these Bushmen supplies a calorie intake variously estimated at 2,260 or 2,140 calories per day during the peak season, with respective estimates for daily protein intake of 93.1 grams or 35 grams (including 2 to 3 grams of animal protein). The Bushmen show no clinical evidence of malnutrition. Interestingly, the women seem to exhibit a seasonal fertility pattern so that pregnancy is most likely to occur during the time when the food supply is greatest.

*Australian Natives Suffer from Civilization*

The Australian aborigines eat from a wide variety of food sources, including wild fruits and vegetables, nuts and seeds, honey, plant gum, flowers, and a variety of animal foods including eggs. They have no definite mealtimes or fixed patterns of eating; the women snack while collecting and the men eat separately when they return from the hunt, sharing some of their meat with the children, then later joining the women and eating the plant foods while the women partake of the animal foods. Robson reports that, based on official American dietary standards, the requirements for certain nutrients are not always met by the aborigines' diet, but the situation becomes much worse when they become settled, with a resultant diminution in the variety of their food intake and the development of such problems as obesity and various medical illnesses.

*Papuans Subsist on Little*

The people of Papua New Guinea eat a diet based on a starchy staple with some secondary foods eaten as side dishes; meat is eaten only rarely in most areas. In some places palm grubs and fish are available, and peanuts, beans, and nuts are also eaten. Daily intake is estimated at 1,300 to 1,900 calories for the lowland dwellers, with crude protein of 10 to 40 grams; in the highlands it is estimated at 1,400 to 2,400 calories, with 20 to 30 grams of protein. The Papua New Guinean diet is universally considered to provide considerably less protein than is generally accepted as necessary to maintain good health. Infants grow relatively slowly during their first nine months of life, when mother's milk is their basic food, and during this period some develop severe malnutrition; but many survive to become strong, healthy adults.

What is the relationship between the diets of these primitive peoples and the state of their health? The ability of certain groups, such as the natives of Papua New Guinea, to survive on much smaller intake of protein than we in the West consider necessary suggests that man is capable of adapting to a wide range of nutrient and calorie intakes. Three possible mechanisms are mentioned by Robson for adaptation to low protein intakes. First, intestinal bacteria in the alimentary canals of the Papua New Guineans appear to synthesize nitrogenous materials from nondietary sources. Second, the Papua New Guineans have a high intake of potassium in the foods they consume, and this seems to result in a saving of protein in the diet through a recycling of metabolic nitrogen. Finally, certain adjustments seem to occur in the metabolic processes in response to low protein intake. Similarly, the body seems to be able to adjust to low caloric intake; what limited evidence there is suggests that the Bushmen, for instance, normally maintain low fasting blood-sugar levels. When hunters and gatherers become acculturated, this adaptive balance is upset and they demonstrate carbohydrate intolerance.

*Man Highly Adaptable*

It has been observed that heart disease and hypertension are rare or absent among primitive peoples, but it is difficult to tell whether this is due to dietary factors or to other causes. Certainly the specific components of the diets of these hunting and gathering groups vary widely, and yet all have certain characteristics in common, such as their relatively small intake of food in proportion to their physical activity. Relatively low blood cholesterol levels have also been observed in the people of Papua New Guinea, as well as in Eskimo groups whose intake of fat is high.

*Heart Disease Rare Among Primitives*

The idea that primitive people do not suffer from cancer because they do not live long enough is a fallacy based on the assumption that low life expectancy is their norm. In fact, the opposite is true. Once these people survive infancy and early childhood, longevity is the norm. The high death rate in premarket societies should be seen as clustered among the very young and the very old.

*Cancer Infrequent*

*Cancer Related to Diet in Industrialized Nations*

Of course, the same inaccurate argument is applied to populations in highly developed societies. We are told by unwise but highly placed scientists, even some Nobel Prize winners, that the reason cancer prevalance is on the rise is because people are now living longer and there are better diagnostic techniques than in the past! Unfortunately, cancer is now a principal cause of death among children, which is definitely a *new* scourge, not due to mere statistical manipulation. In the chapter "Flies in the Slaughterhouse" I very positively identify the food additives that are killing our children, while high sugar, fat, and protein diets as contributors to childhood and adult cancers are examined, with dietary modifications suggested in the chapter "Diet and Cancer."

*Fiber, Sugar, Fats, Significant*

It has been observed that one dietary element that seems to provide protection against cancer is fiber. Fiber in the diet speeds the bowel transit time, so that toxic substances are not in contact with the walls of the intestine for as long; fiber also increases the bowel water content and thus dilutes potential carcinogens. The diet of primitive man contains large quantities of fiber, but there are also other dietary variables that must be considered in their lower incidence of cancer, such as the differences in the quality of the fats ingested, the virtual absence of sucrose in their diets, and the overall low caloric intake. Whatever the reasons—dietary or something else—as these groups become more acculturated, cancer becomes more prevalent among them.

*Disease of Civilization Outlined*

The groups surveyed by Robson have not only been able to survive, sometimes in hostile environments, but they have even been able to increase in population size, collecting sufficient food to sustain strong and active lives once they have survived the first few years of life. Women are able to bear young and nurse them with great efficiency. Obesity, diabetes, high blood pressure, and ischemic heart disease seem to be absent, and the greatest danger to life is not from nutritional deficiencies but rather from infection, which takes a considerable toll among these isolated groups.

# Energy Flow: Primitive and Contemporary

*Ancients in Better Energy Balance*

The reason we have troubled ourselves so with primitive man as a model is because in terms of *energy flow* our ancestors were in better balance than we are. We know from what little evidence there is that the hunter and gatherer, who didn't have to do any work except gather food, spent a relatively small amount of time doing so. He expended very little energy; there was much more energy surrounding him than he had to expend. Food, therefore, was in a markedly positive energy balance.

Later in history, under the primitive slash-and-burn agriculture of the Mayans, it took about seventy-two eight-hour workdays a year to produce enough corn to feed a family of five and the livestock, with enough corn left over to trade. Agriculture was at first a very significant means of capturing the sun's energy and creating a positive energy balance. A study in Guiana has shown that an Indian couple needed to work only ten or twelve weeks in the year, clearing and planting seven or eight acres, to grow sufficient food for a year. The rest of their time remained for pleasure, hunting, and fishing.

We in the United States are very proud of our modern agriculture; we often claim to be the most agriculturally productive country on earth. In terms of energy balance this is absolute and utter nonsense; we are the most wasteful country in the world.

*Mechanized Agriculture Wasteful*

Let's say that one person working alone could produce two units of energy. This means that he could produce more energy than he needed; this would maintain a positive energy flow. Our agriculture, on the other hand, requires about ten units of energy input to produce one unit of energy as food! (The estimates vary from between five to fifteen units in to produce one unit of output.) In our dependence on fossil fuels for the manufacture of fertilizer, putting it on the field, and using machines to till and harvest, we have created an excessive negative energy balance. We have taken the one source of positive energy flow to this planet and completely reversed the process. Our great agriculture has become a destructive force for mankind's future.

Primitive man had a much better food-energy balance than we do; in and of itself that's enough reason to harken back to primitive man as a model. But in addition to energy considerations, we will refer to this important model when we refer again to food, diet, health, and disease, for the purpose of constructing our own diets.

In Anglo-Saxon countries, as Ford Madox Ford once remarked, food is no more talked of than love or Heaven.

—CLIFTON FADIMAN

# 3 THE ETHNIC FACTOR

## Ethnic Diets Adaptive

As our prehistoric ancestors evolved and dispersed through time, there developed a great play and variety of human groups, many now extinct. As diverse as the lands they inhabit, the people of the earth have attempted to control their varied environments in many ingenious ways. This interaction with available resources has given us a tremendous range of ethnic diets.

*Fairly Stable Ethnic Groups Exist*

Intermarriage between widely variant ethnic groups is fairly recent, and constant bloodlines, with fairly stable gene pools, exist even in an age of mass migration and travel. The East Germans, for example, are of fairly constant Teutonic stock; Poles and Yugoslavians descended from the Slavs, while Albanians arrived largely from the Illyrian tribes. Greeks, of course, are not so simply the descendants of any particular group, but derive from many diverse tribes who met and thrived in their islands. Nevertheless, even in Greece a fairly stable ethnic group with a national diet is easily identified. Within Bulgaria, a country shattered by World War II, where great migrations and shifts in population have occurred, there are still clearly defined ethnic groups. We know, for example, that 91 percent of the people are Bulgarians and that Turks make up approximately another 6 percent of the total population. Within this group of Turks two clearly defined groups are found: the Greek-speaking Karakatchans and the Rumanian-speaking Vlachs. Other clearly defined ethnic groups living in Bulgaria include Armenians, Greeks, Gypsies, Jews, Macedonians, Rumanians, and Russians. So, even in an age of great population shifts such as ours, there are highly specific ethnic populations with equally specialized diets suitable for our study.

*Why study ethnic diets?*

It is my belief, based upon medical-anthropological literature and my own travels over a period of a decade, that were we to eat the way our ethnic ancestors did, when food was in abundant supply, we would have much better health. This is not an argument that is readily understood. In our biochemical age doctors have long sought to treat all people as though they were identical biological organisms. Of course, we know how individualized man can be, even our stomachs varying tremendously in anatomical shape. Our needs for specific nutrients have also been shown to vary considerably.* Being as diverse as we are anatomically and in our needs for specific nutrients, might we not be expected to vary even more in our ethnic dietary needs? We are more than mere test tubes, filled with biochemicals. By studying various ethnic diets and their relative nutritional values, we can learn to maximize our health while reestablishing our identities along dietary lines.

*What is this "ethnic factor"?*

Simply this: not everybody can assimilate the same foods in the same way. Depending upon our ethnic, cultural, and religious backgrounds, we utilize foods and respond to fasts differently; these largely psychological factors influence our metabolism in as yet undefined but pronounced ways. Obviously an Alaskan Eskimo is different from a Bantu who is again different from a Yemenite. These differences are both genetic and cultural and translate into varying dietary needs.

*But even if there are ethnic differences in nutrition, where can we find clearly defined ethnic groups in our age of migration and intermarriage?*

As we saw above, the Bulgarian population, for one, is remarkably well defined ethnically. So are populations throughout Eastern Europe, Africa, Asia, and the Pacific. Even in a society as pluralistic as America, specialized pockets of ethnicity remain, surprisingly consistent with earlier dietary patterns. In San Francisco, Vietnamese report that they eat exactly as they did in their country of birth, since the various spices and foodstuffs consumed in Vietnam are readily obtained in Bay Area stores.

*Are you implying that all ethnic diets are inherently wise?*

Not necessarily. The point is that most so-called ethnic diets, as they are presently eaten in Westernized nations, are actually "celebration foods" which were eaten only occasionally in the country of origin. Here, food is in such plentiful supply

---

* See the popular writings of Roger Williams, especially *Nutrition Against Disease.*

that a great distortion in eating habits has occurred. Surely, "Italian" food as prepared in restaurants (even in Italy!) reflects feast days, while also being deficient in many nutrients because of the use of refined flour in preparing pasta, an Old World Italian staple.

*So, by studying our true ethnic diets and applying healthier practices, we will enjoy better balance while reestablishing an important link with our identities?*

Exactly! We are not wed to all dietary items or practices of our ethnic group. Certainly individual preferences based upon familial and individual requirements exist within ethnic groups. By selecting the best of our ethnic foods, we can regain the nutritional balance that was lost during assimilation.

*What about those of us brought up without any particularly strong ethnic identity regarding food?*

For those brought up without any emphatic ethnic dietary patterns, it will be of particular interest to learn about those "ethnic diets" that appeal to us, from a health or culinary point of view. In so doing we gain a deeply sought-after element in our lives, a security about food, associated with the ethnic identities we have "borrowed."

# Diets from the Earth

For the purpose of constructing our own diet, we should look at diets from countries around the world, and trust those elements with obvious health value.

## Oceania

*Heart Disease Not Related to Saturated Fats*

In the Pacific Islands, where one of the most densely saturated vegetable fats is regularly consumed, heart disease is reported as being at particularly low rates. Little has been written regarding the possible relationship between coconuts and heart disease. This important Pacific Island food should be a significant etiological factor in cardiovascular disease if we consider saturated fats as important causal links in coronary artery occlusion. Yet the connection between saturated fats and heart disease may not be so simple after all, for various ethnic groups are able to consume great quantities with apparent impunity. The protein content of coconut cream is both fairly high for a liquid product (4.4 percent) and of good quality—comparable to proteins of pulses, oily seeds, and nuts. The fat content of coconut cream is also high; it is especially rich in saturated fats, while low in the unsaturated fatty acids. Coconut cream contains 28 grams of saturated fatty acids per 100 grams, and only 2 grams of unsaturated fatty acids. Even heavy natural whipped cream, which contains 21 grams of saturated fatty acids per 100 grams, contains 13 grams of unsaturated fatty acids.

By contrast, other vegetable fats used for cooking, which contain 23 grams of saturated fatty acids per 100 grams, contain 72 grams (!) of unsaturated fatty acids. Fresh eggs, often criticizes as being high in saturated fats, contain only 4 grams of saturates and 6 grams of unsaturates per 100 grams.

Furthermore, the relative *balance* between saturated and unsaturated fatty acids gives us an interesting perspective. Coconut cream is ratioed 14:1 (saturates:unsaturates), while milk (human, cow, and goat) is balanced 2:1. Therefore, the balance between saturated and unsaturated fats is severely skewed toward cholesterol-inducing saturated fats for diets rich in coconut cream. If saturated fat is really an etiological factor in coronary heart disease, then why do we find such *low* rates of CHD in indigenous populations where coconut cream is consumed on a regular basis?

The reason why Pacific Islanders who eat traditional diets may be able to eat such a densely saturated fat without suffering a plague of heart attacks is to be found in their intake of other nutrients, from native foods. Roger Williams, the eminent biochemist, makes a strong case for this point of view in his book *Nutrition Against Disease.* He presents many examples of peoples who consume great quantities of saturated fats who have *lower* rates of coronary heart disease than neighboring peoples who consume *low* amounts of saturated fats and correspondingly *high* amounts of polyunsaturated fats. Williams is so convinced of the *negative* relationship between high saturated-fat intake and cardiovascular disease that he reemphasizes this point three times in his book. He offers the hypothesis that those "protected'" groups (who eat a great deal of saturated fats) also eat foods which "are favorable in promoting intestinal synthesis of B vitamins, particularly pyridoxine ($B_6$), which protect against atherosclerosis, and do not create cellular (antioxidant) malnutrition from a too high consumption of polyunsaturated fats." My own studies in the South Pacific Islands and Israel tend to support Williams's hypothesis.

Pacific Island people who still eat a traditional diet of coco-

*Other Nutrients*
*Aid Fat*
*Metabolism*

nut, fish, breadfruit, pandanus, starchy aroids, and their greens receive a good spread of the protective nutrients recommended by Williams, namely, vitamin C, vitamin E, vitamin $B_6$, choline, magnesium, calcium, and trace minerals, with relatively *low* intakes of protein.

Since we are surveying ethnic diets for clues to our own healthful survival, it will be worthwhile to look at some of these Pacific Island foods in greater detail.

*Pacific Island Foods Nutritious*

Pandanus, an important food in Micronesia, contains equal or greater amounts of calcium than white potatoes; about the same amount of phosphorus as fresh fruits; a favorable quantity of iron; more provitamin A than peaches; as good a quantity of thiamine, riboflavin, and niacin as apples, apricots, and pears; and more niacin than is found in sweet potatoes, apples, and pears. These vitamin and calcium values may be extremely important in helping to metabolize dietary fats, especially the highly saturated coconut. Pandanus paste and flour, two "ethnic" preparations, greatly concentrate the amount of calcium available (134 mg/100 g and 797 mg/100 g, respectively).

Breadfruit is another important Pacific Island food, and it too is well endowed with a broad spectrum of vitamins and minerals, with breadfruit paste containing 134 mg of calcium per 100 g.

Taro and other starchy aroids provide the majority of calories in the daily diet of Pacific Islanders. What to the Westerner is just a mass of unappetizing carbohydrate serves these people as a fairly nutritious food. Niacin levels are adequate, as are total calories supplied, and when large amounts of these starchy roots are eaten, as in the habit, they supply a good amount of calcium, phosphorus, and iron.

Interesting from an adaptive point of view is the ethnic dietary wisdom of an ancient Hawaiian "baby formula." The basic constituent, poi (mashed taro), is inadequate infant food by itself, but the people learned to supplement this food with the soft parts of shellfish like opihi (the Hawaiian limpet). This seafood is an excellent source of high-quality protein, and also contains a good supply of riboflavin and vitamin A.

*Cholesterol Levels Unrelated to Hypertension*

Returning to our original search for statistically significant cardiovascular disease rates among various ethnic groups, we might look at two neighboring Polynesian groups living in the Pacific Islands with widely different rates of cardiovascular disease. J. D. Hunter (*Fed. Proc.*, 21, Supp. 11:36, 1962) looked at the Atiu and Mitiaro islanders, who follow a fairly traditional life-style, including diet, and compared them with their Rarotongan neighbors, who are markedly more Europeanized (enjoying a jetport and a continual flow of foreign visitors and imports). As expected, the health effects of modernization are dramatically deleterious regarding hypertension. The traditional group eat a diet rich in highly saturated coconut fat but only 10 percent of these people suffered from hypertension, as compared with 25 percent of the Rarotongan males. Surprisingly, the tradition-bound Atiu-Mitiaro males had serum cholesterol levels as high as those of European males (perhaps from eating coconuts), but electrocardiographic readings did not show any changes that would indicate coronary heart disease. Other dietary factors, such as foods rich in vitamins and minerals, apparently mitigate *against* hypertension. Of course stress levels, sodium intake, physical activity, and patterns of alcohol use and cigarette smoking also influence blood pressure. But for the purposes of this survey dietary factors as such are significant influences.

There are other good studies that tend to support Williams's idea "that adult males of widely differing ethnic stock can subsist on a high fat, high cholesterol, high caloric diet, and yet remain relatively free of cardiovascular disorders." Studies from India, Switzerland, Africa, Alaska, and Roseta, Pennsylvania, all appear to support this hypothesis and are analyzed in detail in Dr. Williams's book, *Nutrition Against Disease.*

Other wisely adaptive indigenous diets may be found worldwide; but for the purposes of this thoughtway I will mention only a few.

## Asia

The betel nut palm *(Areca catechu)* is cultivated widely in Southeast Asia and the Indian subcontinent. Betel nuts wrapped within the leaves of betel pepper *(Piper betel)* and treated with lime are chewed widely in this part of the world, primarily for their stimulant effects. But the nut also contains some calcium. When the betel leaf is treated with lime, as is the custom, the amount of calcium ingested from six betel leaves is comparable to that obtained from 10 ounces of cow's milk.*

---

* Habitual chewers of betel nut have a high incidence of buccal carcinoma, possibly due to the 11 to 26 percent condensed tannins found in the nut. Nevertheless, the addition of lime is a good example of a wise adaptive practice from a nutritional point of view.

*Chinese Dish
Maximizes
Calcium
Absorption*

A typical Chinese dish, sweet-sour spareribs, is prepared with cutup ribs, vinegar, soy sauce, sugar, and salt. The vinegar is wisely added because it helps to transfer much tricalcium phosphate from the bones into the cooking broth. This dish then delivers calcium and phosphorus in abundant amounts.

*Rice Bran Adds
B Vitamins*

Pickled vegetables are widely eaten in Asia. This method was no doubt derived as a means of keeping surplus vegetables from spoiling. But certain components added to the pickling medium profoundly affect the thiamine and niacin values of the vegetables. Chinese cabbage, oriental radish (daikon), and eggplant originally contain only negligible amounts of these B vitamins. As the author of a review article on Asian foods writes: "If pickled with salt alone, some loss of these vitamins occurs. . . . When rice bran is added with the salt the content of thiamine and niacin increases greatly" (Woot-Tsuen Wu Leung, 1964).

*Menus Show
Wisdom*

Other nutritious foods in Asia showing adaptive manipulation include fermented fish sauces (an important source of calcium and protein); shrimp paste (calcium and protein rich); soybean products (tofu, miso, natto, tempeh, etc.); and the leaves and tips of food plants, cooked to eliminate oxalic acid and free dietary calcium.

*Beriberi
Appears Where
Rice Is Milled*

While many diseases related to inadequate food are known in Asia, beriberi is practically unknown wherever *parboiled rice* is used. This wise cooking method retains most thiamine, a critical vitamin for people living close to the edge of starvation. As elsewhere in the world there is a strong relationship between the incidence of beriberi and the distribution of modern rice mills which strip rice of the important bran. Mechanical hullers which mill rice too finely created a situation in Thailand where beriberi ranked tenth among the causes of death (1961). Too thorough milling and the practice of washing rice and then allowing the cooked grains to sit overnight also cause considerable loss of thiamine. Where people retained ancient menus calling for parboiled rice, this dread nutritional disease is practically nonexistent.

## India

This nutritious grain is prepared by soaking rice in cold or lukewarm water for different lengths of time. The grain is then steamed until it becomes soft or partly cooked. Excess water is drained off; the rice paddy is then spread out to dry This parboiled paddy is hulled at this time, leaving grain with its unique appearance and flavor characteristics. Surprisingly, when ready for eating, the grain is slightly colored, and is actually harder to the teeth than the original grain of rice. This ancient practice of parboiling preserves the valuable nutrients to their highest level, particularly vitamin $B_1$, essential in the prevention of beriberi.

Another method of preparing the rice results in a final product which is often used as food for convalescents in India. The paddy is made wet, mixed with about four times its volume of sand that has been preheated in a frying pan, and both items kept together on an open flame. The mixture of rice and sand is stirred rapidly with an iron ladle, and after only a few minutes strained over a wire sieve which retains the rice, letting the sand fall through. The rice at this stage is parched, swollen, and burst, the cracked hull having separated during parching—another delicious, wisely adapted cooking method.

Milk and its by-products are extremely important items of the diet in India, including items such as ghee, butter, buttermilk, and products known as channa, khoa, malai, and rabadi. *Specialized Milk Products Described* Ghee is clarified butter, from which the water has been removed by heating. It is an extremely important food, prepared much like ordinary butter. Milk is brought to a boil and allowed to remain at that boiling temperature for five or more minutes. When it cools to a state of warmth, preformed curd is introduced, resulting in fermentation. An equal quantity of water is added and the mixture is churned in a metallic or clay vessel using a wooden churner. When the butter separates, usually after a half hour, it is removed and pressed. One of the by-products, buttermilk, contains most of the nutrients of fresh milk excluding the fat, and is extremely popular. It is often eaten together with rice; in the north it is drunk. Malai is the cream that has risen to the top of slowly heated milk. Rabadi is simply whole milk that has been boiled down to a thick, syrupy consistency and later sweetened. Khoa is whole milk that has been concentrated in open pans into a state of granular curds which still contain a bit of water; this is the basis of several different Indian sweets. Channa is curdled milk brought to this state by adding rennet or minerals or organic acids. In this poor nation yet greater malnutrition is prevented as a result of these wise methods of food preparation which retain, in fact concentrate, some of the foods' nutrients.

In Western countries, where excess is the rule, fats once avoided like the plague have recently been found "safe" by a *Ethnic Diet May Prevent Heart Disease* committee of the National Academy of Science. But we must remember that fat is only one factor in heart disease, with other factors, of the diet especially, considerably more important. An extremely significant study by Malhotra (1967) compared two groups in India. In the north the diet is rich in milk products, particularly ghee, which has a fat content composed of 45 percent of short-chain fatty acids. In the south, Madras Indians have fifteen times more coronary heart disease, yet consume diets with only 2 percent saturated fats because they are vegetarians! Later surveys showed that northern Indians consume nineteen times more fats than the southern Indians, yet their coronary heart disease rate was as much as fifteen times lower! Obviously, fat in and of itself does not cause atherosclerosis and coronary heart disease. Dr. Roger Williams speculates that

the butter fat and fermented milk drinks common to the northern Indians promote the intestinal flora and presumably the intestinal synthesis of pyridoxine, while the unsaturated fats of the southern Indians need to be accompanied by more pyridoxine in the diet, depress intestinal flora synthesis, and depress calcium absorption. (*Nutrition Against Disease,* p. 300)

Ethnic factors may play a role in heart disease as related to diet, but we would *all* be wise to supplement our diets with 10 to 20 mg of vitamin B$_6$ (pyridoxine) in light of Dr. Williams's remarks.

## Iran

As in India, milk is rarely consumed in its fresh state in Iran. The most commonly used dairy product is yogurt, which in Iran is known as mast. It is either eaten alone, combined with other dishes, or made into a soup which is mixed with cucumbers and seasoned with rose powder and dried raisins. Cheese is also common in Iran, and the type used is a salted white cheese clotted in a pouch that is composed of sheep's stomach. Sheep's or cow's milk is used to prepare this cheese. Butter, as in India, is rarely used fresh but is almost always in the form of a clarified product similar to ghee. While the majority of the people in Iran are living close to a subsistence level and sometimes below it, these few wisely adapted foods spell the difference between total starvation and nutritional diseases. In a country where a majority of the daily diet is cereals, which contribute over 70 percent of the total calories and 66 percent of total proteins, milk products are extremely important in the diet.

## Saudi Arabia

There are three basic types of diets in the Arabian Peninsula: that of the nomadic Bedouin herdsmen, the diet of agriculturists, and the diet of people living in towns and cities. Here again the more traditional diet, that of the Bedouins, is superior. Although they are nomadic, the Bedouins' diet is better balanced nutritionally, even though it is of a lower caloric intake. Some consider the Bedouin diet monotonous, the principal food being milk and milk products of the camel, goat, or sheep. The milk is taken either fresh or in a curdled form similar to yogurt and called laban. Cheese is made from this milk, a type of cream cheese being the most popular. Dates and other dried fruits are eaten from time to time when they can be obtained from settled cultivators. The nomadic Bedouins do eat wheat, barley, and some rice, which is gotten in trade with the agriculturists or occasionally grown by the nomads themselves. Meat is only rarely eaten by the nomadic Bedouins. Only those animals that die of natural causes are eaten because the animal is extremely important in the life of the tribesmen. A central element of the diet, and an extremely important part of the social life of the Bedouins, is coffee, brewed either from the husks or the berry.

*Nomads Enjoy Superior Diet*

The agriculturists in the Arabian Peninsula on first sight appear to eat better. The diet is higher in calories, but deficient in proteins and fats. Grain from millet is used for making flat unleavened bread, and this is augmented by dates, occasional mutton, milk and milk products, fruits and vegetables when available, and some fish. While milk and milk products are certainly available from goats and sheep, surprisingly the consumption is much more limited than among the Bedouins. As with the Bedouins, locusts are considered a delicacy and are eaten—luckily, because they are a good source of high-quality protein.

As elsewhere, urban diets are generally more varied and better nutritionally for those with money. More fresh fruits and vegetables are eaten, more meat is eaten, while the use of dates is less than amongst the Bedouins or the agriculturists. As in all parts of Arabia, women and children eat less and poorer foods than do adult males. It is the universal custom for the father and older sons of the family to eat first, the women and children eating what is left over. Thus women and children often never see foods considered delicacies which are of extreme nutritional importance in a marginal diet, such as meat, fruits, and vegetables, the generally protective foods.

While chronic malnourishment has become a way of life for most inhabitants of Arabia, we see again that a traditional diet amongst the Bedouins is often the wisest nutritionally, while low in calories.

## Israel

*Yemenite Diet Wise*

Proponents of an increased intake of raw foods or a total raw food diet will find interest in the Yemenite people of Israel. Yemeni Jews have a rather limited diet characterized by the fact that little cooking is done. Intake of fats is lower than the Israeli average, the number of calories is lower, and this is all related to the fact that Yemenites do not drink milk, use any spreads on bread, or eat cheese. Dishes such as houmous (mashed chickpeas) and many different vegetable dishes are popular amongst the Yemenite people, and have been accepted rapidly into Israeli society. For the purpose of this brief survey of various ethnic cuisines of the world with dietary wisdom, the Yemenites are the most interesting group in Israel. Some people consider this group more representative of an authentic ancient Israelite nation. Jews from Palestine settled in what is now known as Saudi Arabia shortly after the destruction of the Second Temple. For several thousand years they lived in this diaspora in a manner not totally dissimilar to the one they left behind. Consequently, their diet may be more representative of a "traditional" Jewish diet.

Interestingly, part of the folklore of this group of people contained the belief that one day God would send a gigantic bird from the sky to lift them up and bring them back to their promised land from which they had been exiled, and this dream was fulfilled when shortly after the creation of the Jewish state the Israeli government sent several cargo planes and airlifted the entire persecuted Yemenite Jewish community en masse to Israel.

*Fava Beans Deadly to Some*

A smaller group of Jewish people from Habban, Southern Arabia, emigrated to Israel shortly after 1948, and have been living as a very closed community within Israeli society. Their population consists of only four lineages, totaling approximately 1,250 people. The number of marriages and matings of close relatives is very high among the Habbanites (56 percent), many of these being first-cousin marriages, and these people have been studied very carefully from a genetic point of view. Certain rare genetic disorders occur in this close-knit community; however, we are concerned with nutrition-related problems only. Fava bean hemolysis is quite prevalent amongst these people and other Oriental Jewish groups, the Kurds having one of the highest frequencies of this disorder on record. Favism affects individuals with a Mediterranean phenotype, and hemolysis can occur within only a few hours of inhaling pollen of fava bean plants, or within one or two days after eating fresh or dried fava beans. The urine becomes very dark or red, shock may develop in bad cases, and death can follow. This condition is caused by a lack of glucose-6-phosphate dehydrogenase (G6PD).

Knowledge of the toxic responses of individuals with this deficiency dates back to antiquity. As far back as Pythagoras in the sixth century B.C., people were warned that eating this type of bean could yield death, while in the fifth century B.C., Herodotus also mentioned favism. In this century acute hemolytic anemia was first reported in 1926 in a Panamanian plantation population who had received the drug called Plasmochin during their treatment for malaria. It seems that this drug was capable of inducing this severe form of anemia. While G6PD deficiency is most severe in the Mediterranean populations, and hemolytic anemia occurs most frequently amongst this population, it can also occur in other people. As a result certain drugs and chemicals being administered—drugs such as acetanilid, chloramphenicol, naphthalene, pamaquine, primaquine, quinidine, sulfanilamide—are all capable of bringing about hemolytic reactions in G6PD-deficient people. When acute hemolytic anemia is induced, abdominal or back pain often occurs, the urine can turn dark, even black, and then signs of erythrocyte regeneration appear. Thus even an important stable food such as the fava bean can be deadly to those individuals with a genetic deficiency. Here is another example of the classic "one man's meat is another's poison." We can all learn from this, and remember not to admonish our friends who may find some of our most magical food combinations totally repugnant. This abhorrence for our favorite food can often reflect a survival instinct which we must learn to respect.

For those who like statistics, it may be interesting to note that this G6PD deficiency in the non-Ashkenazi (non-European) population of Israel varies from 1 percent to 2 percent among European Sephardim, up to 25 percent among Iraqi Jews, 28 percent among Caucasus Jews examined, and over 61 percent among Kurdish Jews. Of the Arabs studied, just a bit over 4 percent of the people exhibited this deficiency. In the southern Sinai, only 2 percent of the Towara Bedouins exhibited this deficiency, while up to 20 percent of those studied amongst the Mamassani tribespeople of Iran and 21.4 percent of people in Kuwait studied showed it, while the Druses and Armenians of Lebanon exhibited o percent. This fascinating study, and countless others, are all contained in a master medical work written by Dr. Richard M. Goodman entitled *Genetic Disorders Among the Jewish People.*

*Diabetes Rates Rise as Diet Shifts*

An example of disease states that can be induced as a result of severe and dramatic dietary changes can be found amongst the Yemenite Jewish people. For example, the Kurds and Yemenites who came to Israel had rates of diabetes as low as the Eskimos of Iceland and Greenland (0.3 per 1,000). Both groups lived in an isolated geographical situation, with little contact with Western life-style including diet. Soon after settling in areas where Western habits and diets prevail, a sharp rise in the prevalence of diabetes is noted. This is held up by a study done by A. M. Cohen in 1958, who compared the rates of occurrence in four Jewish ethnic groups in Israel, based on the father's place of birth. These were Sephardic, Ashkenazi, Yemenite, and Kurdish communities. The study sample was composed of nearly 16 thousand people, half males and half females, and their age distribution resembled that of the general Israeli population. Interestingly, the lowest rates of diabetes mellitus were seen among Yemenite newcomers (0.06 percent), followed by the Sephardic people (1 percent), while the old Yemenite settlers had the highest rate (2.9 percent), even higher than that of Ashkenazi Jews (2.5 percent). Dr. Goodman cites an animal experiment conducted in 1964 by Schmidt-Nielsen in which sand rats were transferred

from their natural desert habitat to a laboratory environment. The rats that were transferred and their first generation offspring exhibited inappropriate hyperglycemia associated with obesity and diabetes. Subsequent generations tended to adapt to laboratory conditions and displayed mild or no hyperglycemia. In man, however, these adaptations do not occur as readily, as evidenced by the higher rate of diabetes among second-generation Israelis.

*Refined Carbohydrates Implicated in Diabetes*

Some think that obesity and diabetes indicate a failure to adapt to rapid changes in life-style, both in sand rats and people. From my point of view, dietary changes are more important. A visit to Israel will show constant feeding upon coffee and sweets at all times of day and late into the evening. Yes, genetic factors may play a role in diabetes and other diseases, because we do know that certain ethnic groups have a high rate of diabetes mellitus, especially different American Indian tribes and certain tribes in South Africa; but even these groups must be looked at in the context of total life-style change, including dietary consumption of refined carbohydrates.

## Africa

SENEGAL   In a continent of malnutrition, some peoples live very good lives, due in part to luck of geography, but also because they know how to combine the foods of their land. One of the best diets on the continent is found amongst the Toucouleurs of the middle Senegal valley. The diet is primarily based on cereals, milk, and fish. Amongst the cereals, millet and sorghum supply the energy, milk and fish supply proteins and minerals, while vitamin A is supplied by leaves, cereals, and milk. Riboflavin, while not adequately supplied, comes from milk and fish, and the limiting amino acid in the diet is methionine. Interestingly, there is an inadequate amount of vitamin C in the diet, mainly from milk and leaves. These Africans show a minimal amount of nutritional deficiencies, except for a xerophthalmia (dryness of conjunctiva and cornea due to vitamin A deficiency), which is seasonal in character, disappearing during the mango season.

A related people, the Diolas of the Casamance River basin, eat rice mixed with beans, oysters, and fish, occasionally taking millet, sorghum, and tubers. Interestingly, amongst these people many children and pregnant women eat earth to compensate for mineral deficiencies—another example of an intuitive dietary addition.

THE CONGO   Looking at tribal diets amongst the Congolese, we find that the most influential factor in determining what is eaten is not the environment, because there are neighboring tribes with almost completely different diets and who live in almost identical environments. The tribe known as Kuba enjoys one of the best lives of all in the Congo. They produce more than they need, and are agriculturists. They eat corn, manioc, beans, ground nuts and peas, with animal proteins coming from ants, caterpillars, fish, mollusks, and game. Salt is made from plants treated with hot water. The excess products are sold on the market. An adjacent tribe, the Lele, lives a very mediocre existence. These people inhabit very poor soil. While their land area is rich in streams and rivers, with much

*Some Groups Better Nutritionists*

water life, they are very poor fishermen, and their catch is meager. In other parts of the Congo, caterpillars are an important source of animal protein. The Bolendas, for example, do not fish or hunt. They feed on mushrooms, green leaves, roots, and oil, and during the caterpillar season, which lasts three months, this food is their main occupation. While an average mushroom meal gives them about 750 calories, if caterpillars are added, they gain 2,200 calories in a typical meal.

The Pygmies are also found in the Congo. While there is a popular notion that they hunt elephants and bring them down in abundant supply, their diet consists primarily of plantain and fruit.

An important component of dishes in the Congo are the salted fluids that are made from salt-rich leaves. These mineral-rich vegetables include such salt-containing plants as Scleria species, and other plants such as the lotus. Such leaves as these are heated until they are charred, and the resulting ash placed in a filter, water then being poured over it. The resulting salty fluid is used in many different ways.

Throughout the Congo various fermented beverages are prepared, palm wine being one of the most popular beverages. This wine is derived from the sap of the palm tree which has spontaneously fermented, but occasionally fermentation is induced by adding a few vegetable products. Other fermented beverages are made from the pineapple or from sugarcane, while a native beer is made from manioc flour. As elsewhere in the world, an occasional escape from the vicissitudes of life is very much a part of nutrition. We can even argue that without this escape an otherwise difficult life would be totally intolerable.

*Food Taboos Diminish Health*

GHANA  In this country we see an example of poor nutrition within a tribal setting. Here is where bioclimatic conditions and traditions which are negative from a nutritional standpoint actually diminish already meager resources. Taboos such as those against eggs for women and first-born sons in the north of Ghana actually deprive these segments of the population of their access to first-rate proteins. In looking at this taboo, we must ask ourselves how many of our habits of food prohibitions and food choices are based on taboos, traditional or contemporary, which may be depriving us of better health.

NIGERIA  While malnutrition is as common in Nigeria as elsewhere in Africa, starvation is not more widespread because of a few cooking tricks developed through time. Manioc, which contains some degree of cyanogenetic glycosides which can be toxic, is a staple food in this country and elsewhere in the world, but through trial and error the people have found that by drying and grating it becomes a palatable, nutritious food. In Nigeria this root crop is augmented with kola nuts, which are eaten like candy, and occasionally rice, yams, beans, ground nuts, and corn. Fortunately the soups made in this part of the world always contain ground locust bean cakes, which have a good amount of vegetable protein, and palm oil, an extremely important source of vitamin A, salt which contains minerals, and pepper as a flavoring. The soup is often thickened with several ingredients including dried baobob leaves, dried okra, or powdered melon seed, the later being a rich protein source. According to Jacques M. May, while a "wide variety of foods is available in Nigeria the diets are astonishingly monotonous and self limited." Fruit is available widely, but hardly consumed at all. Fats, also widely available from vegetable sources, are not widely eaten.

As elsewhere, as soon as a Nigerian rises on the social scale, the quality and the quantity of food improve. People do not live on meager diets out of moral choice, nor do they elect out of moral choice to attend expensive clinics in Beverly Hills and pay $5,000 for the privilege of living on a starvation diet in the hope that somehow their longevity will be benefited. One disastrous result of acculturation in Nigeria is the elimination of breast-feeding in favor of the more stylish bottle-feeding. Unfortunately for the poor Nigerian women and infants, especially in the rural areas where sterile water, refrigeration, and boiled bottles are hardly available, infant diarrhea is often quite severe. In addition, cow's milk is certainly no competitor for mother's milk, the perfect infant formula.

*Social Position and Foods Related*

## Ethnic Dietary Wisdom

These few examples of wisely adaptive ethnic foods serve to demonstrate two major points. One, health can be maximized and the risk of developing several major nutrition-related diseases lessened by eating in accordance with time-tested foods and food combinations, and by eating *less!* Second, underdeveloped nations whose diets have not been acculturated are generally more highly advanced in terms of adaptive recipes than "developed" nations. That is, their foods are less costly to produce in the overall scheme of energy exchange while adaptations (such as the corn-and-beans combination in Mexico) provide complete proteins without utilizing the flesh of animals, wherever possible. In China, as we saw, the traditional diet for thousands of years has emphasized grains because it is obviously "more economical to feed people with the plants that grow in the soil rather than to depend upon animals to convert the plants into the nutrients needed by man" (Chang, 1977).

## Cancer and Culture

There are wide variations in the incidence of cancer among different cultures, even when groups of relatively similar ethnic background are considered. These differences can often be explained on the basis of environmental factors, including diet, and are generally *not* racial or genetic in origin (see Higginson, 1968). While the topic of cancer and diet is expanded in some detail in a later chapter, a few examples here will serve to show how inherent dietary wisdom protects some groups and a lack of this wisdom proves fatal to others. We must look to these examples when calculating our own nutritional needs.

*Some Cancers Related to Diet*

In the Gonbad region of Iran, for example, the incidence of esophageal cancer is among the highest in the entire world. The diet is simple but lacks protective amounts of vitamin A, vitamin C, and riboflavin. Mozambique has the world's highest known incidence of liver cancer, owing to the ingestion of aflatoxins, a naturally occurring contaminant found largely in nuts and other important vegetable proteins. Seventh-Day Adventists in the United States abstain from smoking and drinking, use fewer processed and refined foods than the general American population, eat high-fiber, low-fat, and low-cholesterol foods, have high intakes of vitamins A and C, and otherwise exhibit a remarkable dietary wisdom. Consequently their mortality rates for cancer is only 50 to 70 percent of the general population.

*Hot Foods Unwise*

Stomach cancer in Japan is still an important cause of suffering and death. There are many theories to account for this, such as the frequent taking of hot tea, wood splinters from inexpensive chopsticks, the presence of asbestos powder in the talc used to coat rice, and so on.* The fact that women have a significantly *lower* rate of this dread disease can be explained by a simple observation often completely overlooked by epide-

---

* Creosote, a potent carcinogen, is a major component of a very popular home-remedy for stomach-ache in Japan. Yet this product has not yet been evaluated as a contributing factor in stomach cancer. The author and his colleague, Dr. Sheldon Margen, are pursuing this line of research as this manuscript goes to press.

miologists. Since women still observe the custom of serving meals to others in the household *before* they themselves eat, it seems to me that food and drink would be *less hot* by the time the women eat, and therefore less likely to irritate delicate tissues. The drop in temperature of a steaming dish, just off the flame, is dramatic within just a few minutes. This circumstantial evidence leads me to recommend the age-old tenet to take food that is neither too hot nor too cold.

I use a simple method to gauge the temperature of hot liquids. My mouth has been conditioned to hot food for so many years that I rarely feel heat with my tongue, lips, or buccal sensors anymore. But by dipping my fingertip into hot drinks, I can *feel* with intensity what a near-boiling liquid must do to my poor innards. Only when the liquid feels comfortably warm to my fingertip do I drink it.

Thus there *are* differences of disease rates where dietary factors play a role, and we *can* control our health to a greater degree than most physicians will admit. And we will soon see how to devise our own plan for doing so.

Unlike science, which *demands* skepticism, religion rests on a "willing suspension of disbelief."

# 4
# ETHNIC DIETS FROM THE DISTANT PAST

Biologically, we are still simple tribal animals: the plant, berry, and occasional flesh-eaters described earlier. But how we went from this free-roaming state, where we received all necessary nutrients, to our present example of vitamin/mineral super-dosers, has never been adequately explained. True, our essentially exploratory, inventive brain likes to play with new techniques, including a simplified method of receiving nourishment. While pills may technically satisfy some of our strictly nutritional needs, and be a signpost of the future where all ethnic dietary difference will have been eradicated by corporate and population pressures, I prefer the canoe to the starship, and choose to live with my body as it is created. We are *not* one hair different from our distant ancestors, physiologically, and we therefore need to try and reconstruct diets of approximately one thousand to four thousand years back if our look at "Diets from the Earth" is to have any relative meaning.

## Ancient Greece

It is worthwhile to pause and study "A Picture of Primitive Life" as described in Plato's *Republic,* for it contains a portrait of an idealized ancient Greek diet type:

*Simple Diet Emphasized*

"Will they not produce corn, and wine, and clothes, and shoes, and build houses for themselves? . . . They will feed on barley-meal and flour of wheat, baking and kneading them, making noble cakes and loaves. . . . And they and their children will feast, drinking of the wine which they have made, wearing garlands on their heads, and hymning the praises of the gods, in happy converse with one another. . . ."

"But," said Glaucon, interposing, "you have not given them a relish to their meal."

"True," I replied, "I had forgotten; of course they must have a relish—salt, and olives, and cheese and they will boil roots and herbs such as country people prepare; for a dessert we shall give them figs, and peas, and beans; and they will roast myrtle-berries and acorns at the fire, drinking, in moderation. And with such a diet they may be expected to live in peace and health to a good old age, and bequeath a similar life to their children after them." (pp. 64–65)

These simple foods would provide a perfectly adequate nutritional base, and might serve as a model for those wanting to adopt a classic Mediterranean diet.

# Ancient China

An early medical writer, Sun Ssemiao (sixth century, A.D.), says: "A true doctor first finds out the cause of the disease, and having found that out, he tries to cure it first by food. When food fails, then he prescribes medicine." Thus we find the earliest existing Chinese book on food, written by an Imperial physician at the Mongol Court in 1330, regards food essentially as a matter of regimen for health, and makes the introductory remarks: "He who would take good care of his health should be sparing in his tastes, banish his worries, temper his desires, restrain his emotions, take good care of his vital force, spare his words, regard lightly success and failure, ignore sorrows and difficulties, drive away foolish ambitions, avoid great likes and dislikes, calm his vision and his hearing, and be faithful in his internal regimen. How can one have sickness if he does not tire his spirits and worry his soul? Therefore he who would nourish his nature should eat only when he is hungry and not fill himself with food, and he should drink only when he is thirsty and not fill himself with too much drink. He should eat little and between long intervals, and not too much and too constantly. He should aim at being a little hungry when well-filled, and being a little well-filled when hungry. Being well-filled hurts the lungs and being hungry hurts the flow of vital energy." (Lin Yutang, *The Importance of Living*)

K. C. Chang lists foods of ancient China in his richly edited text, *Food in Chinese Culture.* We learn that "quantitative data are not available" for this period and that "the following enumeration is highly impressionistic":

Starch Staples: millet, rice, *Kao-liang,* wheat, maize, buckwheat, yam, sweet potato.

Legumes: soybean, broad bean, peanut, mung bean.

Vegetables: malva, amaranth, Chinese cabbage, mustard green, turnip, radish, mushroom.

Fruits: peach, apricot, plum, apple, jujube date, pear, crab apple, mountain haw, longan, litchi, orange.

Meats: pork, dog, beef, mutton, venison, chicken, duck, goose, pheasant, many fishes.

Spices: red pepper, ginger, garlic, spring onion, cinnamon.

Chang emphasizes that the above list has been subject to change, through time. Foreign foods have been brought into China since early times—wheat, sheep, and goat from western Asia; a wide variety of fruits and vegetables from central Asia; sweet potatoes and peanuts from "coastal traders during the Ming period." While all these introductions became integrated into Chinese menus, milk and dairy products, which were introduced in early historical times, have never been widely adopted by the Chinese people. We learn that "this selectivity can be accounted for only in terms of the indigenous cultural base which absorbs or rejects foreign imports according to their structural or stylistic compatibility."

*Our Attitudes in Flux*

We are presently going through a similar period of intense reevaluation, where all of our foods, diet types, menus, food quantity, and internal cleanliness are open to question. It remains to be seen how *our* "cultural base," which is largely composed of medieval northern European and puritanical elements, will influence the selection process. Our diets are in flux and we can only hope to influence the great corporate technology that threatens to drown our sweetest and wisest approach to diet and health. This ancient Chinese food list will become an important reference when we construct our own health plan.

# Maimonides's Views on Health and Nutrition

It is now fairly well appreciated that in ancient texts the diet was first modified during illness; that is, a patient was treated first through food. When this failed to effect a cure, then medicines were tried. Having researched some ancient medical writings, I have found that there are dietary principles which are universally applicable. While these principles are contained in the ancient Chinese, Greek, and Hebrew literature, they are perhaps best stated in the writings of the twelfth-century Jewish physician and scholar, Rabbi Moses Ben Maimon, known as Maimonides. The following excerpts from his *Book of Knowledge* are sound approaches to food and nutrition. He offers much wise advice regarding the total context of food and dietetics, including exercise, excretion, sexuality, moral climate, bathing, and many other elements in his code for physical well-being. This early healer antedates the present school of "holistic" medicine. In those days the whole was not stripped of its component parts, to be sold piecemeal to a fragmented public.

"The first rule regarding food is that one should not eat except when one is hungry, nor drink unless one is thirsty." The second most important rule, that regarding elimination, is that "one should not neglect the calls of nature for a single moment, but respond to them immediately." If we were to follow just these two simple rules, many of our problems would be solved.

Some other general dietary rules are as follows:

*Eat Two-Thirds of What You Can Hold*

Food should not be taken to repletion. During a meal about one third less should be eaten than the quantity that would give a feeling of satiety, and only a little water should be drunk, and that mixed with wine. No meal should be taken without previously walking till the body begins to get warm, or engaging in some kind of exercise or labor; in short, some form of strenuous exercise should be taken daily in the morning, until the body is in a roseate glow. Then there should be an interval of rest till one has recovered composure. If one has the time the exercise can be followed by a bath of warm water, and then a rest before the meal. Before eating careful attention should be paid to the functions of excretion.

As stated in a wise translation of Maimonides, "one should ascertain if they have the urge to purge."

The ancients often advised that one should sit or recline on the left side during a meal. While this is no longer possible, the other associated corollary can certainly be practiced. That is, "One should not walk, ride, take violent exercise, sway the body, or engage in sport, until the food is somewhat digested." It was felt that anyone who engaged in sport or violent exercise

*Restful Attitude Advised*

immediately after a meal subjected himself to grave disorders. Another early precept regarding food and diet advises that one should not sleep immediately after a meal, but only when three or four hours have elapsed. A walk is generally advised following food.

It is advised that laxative foods, such as grapes, figs, mulberries, pears, watermelons, the various kinds of cucumbers or gherkins, should be eaten before a meal. These however should not be mixed with the main dish constituting the meal. After a brief rest, during which these laxative foods have passed out of the stomach, the main meal is eaten. It is recommended that immediately after the meal, foods that tone up the digestive organs should be eaten, such as pomegranates, quinces, apples, and small pears, but even these fruits must not be indulged in too freely.

*Cold Foods in Summer*

Seasonality was also an important part of ancient dietetics. It was advised that "in the summertime cold food should be consumed, and that one should be very sparing with hot spices and condiments." Vinegar was recommended in the summer. During winter warm foods were advised, and condiments were thought to be beneficial when liberally used. It was also advised that similar plans be followed in cold and warm countries. An early ecological approach to nutrition suggested that the diet in every district should be chosen to suit the climate.

*Avoid Stale, Salty, or Preserved Food*

While specific dietary prohibitions of specific foods may not be appropriately listed here, the principles behind these prohibitions may be useful. In looking through the list, it is apparent that stale food is to be avoided, salted food is to avoided, cooked food that has been kept so long that it has lost its savor is to be avoided, any food that is malodorous or very bitter, "all these are like deadly poison to the body." Other foods which are advised *not* to be eaten on a regular basis, but only on occasion, include "large fish, all salty cheeses, too fresh milk, the meat of large animals." (It is interesting to note that large fish contain more methyl mercury than small fish; this was true even in ancient days, since mercury is found naturally in the oceans.) Other foods to be avoided:

. . . those that are considered bad but not to the extent of those just mentioned, include any kind of meal so completely sifted that not a trace of bran remains in it, the blood of meat, gravies, the brine of salted fish, or any kind of bread fried in oil, or the dough of which is kneeded in oil. These can be eaten on an occasional basis, but should not be freely used.

Surprisingly, caution is offered regarding fruits, whether fresh or dried. While figs, grapes, and almonds, whether fresh or dried, are recommended to be eaten "as much as one needs, but not exclusively," an argument is proposed *against* the fruitarian diet. Interestingly, honey and wine are said to be "bad for young children, but good for the aged, particularly in the winter." We are advised that the quantity taken in the summer should be two-thirds of that consumed in the winter. (It is interesting that raw honey has recently been named as a potential source of the causative organisms responsible for sudden infant death.)

It has always been a leading principle in medicine—right up until modern times, when it seems to have been forgotten—that if there is constipation or if the bowels move with difficulty, grave disorders result, and that it should be

*"Do Not Resist the Urge to Purge"*

everyone's care to secure free action of the bowels approximating a relaxed condition. How is a slight costive condition to be remedied? If the patient is young, he should eat every morning salty foods, well cooked and seasoned with olive oil, salt water without bread, or he should drink the liquid of boiled spinach mixed with olive oil and salty water. It is recommended that an old man who is constipated drink in the morning honey diluted with warm water and wait about four hours before taking his breakfast. This regimen should be observed for one day, or if necessary for three or four successive days until the bowels move freely.

Another great principle of health passed on by Maimonides is as follows:

*Even Good Food Harmful If Overeaten*

As long as a person takes active exercise, works hard, does not overeat, and keeps his bowels open, he will be free from disease, and will increase in vigor, even though the food he eats is simple and coarse. But if one leads a sedentary life, and does not take exercise, neglects the calls of nature and is constipated, even if he eats wholesome food and takes care of himself in accordance with medical rules, he will throughout his life be subject to aches and pains and his strength will fail him. It has been said that overeating is like a deadly poison to any constitution, and is the principal cause of all diseases. Most maladies that afflict mankind are thought to result from bad food, or are due to the patient filling his stomach with an excess of food that may even have been wholesome. Thus, Solomon in his wisdom said, "He who keeps his mouth and tongue keeps his soul from troubles" (Prov. 21:23). This text can be applied both to guarding one's mouth from overeating and eating bad food, and from speaking excessively.

# Ancient Mexico and Central America

Beans and corn have been eaten together since antiquity in Mesoamerica and the Andean region. But traditional dietary combinations are not the result of chance. In the case of the corn-and-beans diet, this evolved slowly by "sampling the vegetation over a period of perhaps 1,400 to 3,000 years prior to the establishment of corn and beans agriculture, roughly 6,000 years ago in Middle America. . . . Given sufficient time, a comparable biota, and similar human practices, the same plants would probably be domesticated all over again" (Kaplan, 1969). This useful combination is a matter of survival, owing to the incompleteness of the proteins in each plant food alone. When eaten together, a complete protein made up of all essential amino acids results.

*Dietary Wisdom Takes Much Trial*

It took three thousand years to devise this combination, yet we attempt to combine foods, supplements, and medicines in a wisely adaptive way over a period of only a few years! And with potentially disastrous results: diseases as yet unfound may appear ten, twenty, or thirty years down the line!

Analysis of corn and beans eaten by contemporary Yucatecan Indians shows that the principal corn protein, zein, complements the alpha and beta globulins of black beans. Corn is *always* deficient in two essential amino acids, tryptophane and lysine, while beans "of different varieties and even of different *Phaseolus* species are moderately *high* in lysine and tryptophane." By combining the two foods, early agricultural peoples wisely achieved a dietary protein of high biological value. Here is another example of ethnic dietary wisdom.

# Too Many Wells of Health

*Recreational Healing chastised*

While all peoples have attempted to devise patterns to promote health and longevity, we in the Western world seem to be sampling from all modes at once. It is as though we are walking on a beach in a region noted for its aged, healthful residents. Stopping the first graybeard, his eyes smiling, as he plays with his three small dogs, we learn that his "secret" is a half pint of vodka every day for the past sixty of his eighty years. Making a mental note to switch from wine to vodka, and to drink without guilt from that moment on (!), we continue our walk in the winter sun, coming upon a healthy aged lady doing her T'ai Chi. Incorporating *that* technique in our list of rules for health and longevity, we notice that farther along a crowd has gathered, cheerfully welcoming another hardy octogenarian coming in from his daily swim in the winter sea. We promise ourselves that each day we will religiously swim two miles in the ocean, do our T'ai Chi, drink our half pint of vodka, take our vitamins, have more sex, worry less, pray more (we learned from another resident that 4:00 A.M. prayer was *his* secret), eat six small meals instead of three large ones, get "bodywork," meditate, keep a journal, listen to "clearing" music, etcetera and so on.

Now, while each of these activities (or disciplines of inaction) may have a kernel of wisdom, *all* together must run at cross purposes. Similarly, we *cannot* expect a mélange of menus to yield more than a gustatorial mess, nor can we hope to find our way by employing every little health secret in a random manner. Never mind that current enthusiasm for running madly through traffic or around reservoirs; sitting pleasantly in the sun feeding pigeons may be better for your arteries! Likewise with your own already established dietary patterns.

By all means experiment and enjoy your sampling of "foreign" recipes. But realize that you may have individual dietary needs, some apparent already—what are your cravings; which foods give you a rash; and so on—and some which can only be determined by proper clinical analysis.* Trust your instincts and your stomach; in conjunction with the computer and the laboratory, they can give you a fairly good map of your inner world.

*Limit Your
Food Selections*

# Religion, Ritual, Food, and Health

Mere animals simply eat. As fundamentally *spiritual* creatures we often surround our food and eating habits with rituals and restrictions that very strongly influence our well-being. The effect of religion on our eating habits has been tremendous. The starts and stops of food prohibitions have reshaped our minds, if not our bodies. Eat this, avoid that; on such-and-such a day do not eat at all. Remember to say these words before eating and those words after eating. Having cerebralized our eating habits, religion paved the way for the present generation of approach-avoidance eaters. We have long been condi-

* Discussed in detail in Chapter 12, "At the Nutritionist's."

tioned to *avoid* some perfectly nutritious foods. As a mark of self-discipline we now enjoy rejecting eggs, fatty meats and dairy products, sugar, salt, and additives. The groundwork in rejection and constraint having been laid five thousand years ago, we have recently rediscovered the pleasure and the power of rejecting with gusto.

*Diet* Not *Cause of all Disease*

I am convinced that *without* some form of resistance to certain foods (i.e., food prohibitions or "taboos"), man is very uncomfortable. Our present concern with diet, a bizarre rush to find a dietary culprit for *all* of man's ills and pains, is one road to madness. Yet like many madnesses this hypothesis presents a kernel of essential truth. Diet and behavioral ritual *are* interrelated and affect our health, but not solely in pathways explained by physiology.

*Need to Resist*

By resisting we grow strong, whatever pleasure it is we resist! Like it or not, this is a basic tenet of the world's chief religions. Self-denial is associated with strength, and the kingdom of food is not to be omitted from things resistable. Precisely *what* we must resist is as much a reflection of practical wisdom or commonsense observation as it is a reflection of resistance for the sake of resistance, with cultural and religious bias influencing our choices.

Pork is taboo to many of the world's peoples, yet not all religions that proscribe pork also proscribe shellfish, as do the Jewish dietary laws. Why these bottom-feeding sea creatures were cast from early Hebrew tables has good foundation in commonsense observation. Perhaps the early biblical writers* observed that those who ate shellfish were more often ill than those who abstained. In areas where hygienic measures are lax, seafood poisoning is still a major medical problem, but there are more subtle reasons for avoiding or greatly restricting the consumption of shellfish.

Oysters, for example, can carry copper concentrations as high as 200 to 400 parts per million. Whole grains, as a comparison, contain only 4 to 6 parts per million, while 10 parts per million per day is the concentration normally present in a typi-

---

* Those who ascribe all five books of the Old Testament to divine origin can safely skip this section. My belief in God does not forbid me from believing that early health sanitarians prohibited pork and shellfish solely for hygienic reasons, and that it was men who wrote some laws, especially those dealing with food. The argument that the biblical diet laws were given to us as an ethical system hold water insofar as they limit blood lust when slaughtering higher animals is concerned. When it comes to shellfish, though, there is absolutely no ethical reason to explain this prohibition. It makes sense only from a hygienic point of view.

cal human diet. Why worry about copper from seafood? Because, if we accept the theory of Dr. Carl Pfeiffer ("Mental and Elemental Nutrients"), elevated copper levels often explain the severe depression of many people.

Interestingly, several days prior to menstruation some women have greatly elevated copper levels, which may explain why they "feel like climbing the walls," or "act like witches." I often recommend 30 mg of zinc once daily for three days prior to menstruation, for many of my female clients, with a great deal of success. Symptoms of premenstrual tension and depression appear to be lessened by this copper-zinc interaction, perhaps owing to a protection against the minor copper toxicosis which sometimes occurs.

*Zinc Relieves Premenstrual Tension*

These few examples of the potential hazards of shellfish are included to encourage us not to be too quick to scorn the possible validity of the Hebrew Scriptures' prohibition against eating these creatures. Religious dietary laws may not always make sense to us, but they were carefully evolved through time and can sometimes be explained on a purely rational medical level. When evaluating various ethnic diets from around the world for clues to *your* optimal diet, pay particular attention to the cultural and religious framework in which the menus are eaten. They may have some useful purpose in as yet undetermined pathways.

*Diets Are Part of Greater Framework*

We are more than *what* we eat. We are also *how* we eat, *when* we eat, and what we leave behind, not mere bags within bags of protoplasm to be adjusted by simple biochemical manipulations. *Food is intricately interwoven with our souls.*

# Book Two
## DAWN LIGHT

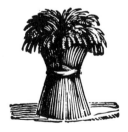

# 5 OVERCOMING THE FAMINE WITHIN

Just as the bear knows which plants to eat when sick, the ancients and contemporary primitives seek the calm and the cure from the earth. People have tried to find the path to health and longevity since the beginning, apparently supplementing their diets with vitamin/mineral-rich infusions and decoctions as well as with concentrated foods (such as crushed oyster or eggshells, bones, or plant ash), and via the intensive nutrition associated with specialized recipes (such as dishes of brains, kidneys, thymus, and intestine). These dietary supplements are variously rich reservoirs of many vitamins and minerals, as well as of high-quality protein. Many skeptics will say that we do *not* need supplements, because our ancestors never took them and they are new to nature. What I hope to demonstrate is that supplementation has been practiced since antiquity, in the forms just mentioned.

*Supplements Taken Since Antiquity*

## Vitamin/Mineral Supplementation: An Ancient Theme

Supplementation in antiquity with various nutritious items (plants, animals, and minerals) has generally been overlooked on the assumption that traditional diets were already nutrient rich. My decade of investigations in Fiji and Tonga and a review of the literature has led me to conclude that *intensive supplementation* has long been practiced and on a fairly regular basis, especially when the slightest everyday complaint is experienced—contrary to current romantic notions of the stoicism of primitive peoples! Headaches, stomachaches, sniffles, aches and pains, insomnia, fright, diarrhea, constipation, loss of appe-

*Folk Remedies Rich Source of Vitamins*

49

tite, and other "minor" complaints, the "many sins that flesh is heir to," are generally treated with vitamin- and mineral-rich remedies in primitive cultures.

While some remedies are of doubtful medicinal efficacy, all plant medicines contain some nutrients and are to be considered dietary adjuncts. Since most plant remedies are prepared as warm-water infusions, vitamins and minerals are extracted and consumed, not being lost to heat as by some cooking methods.

*Specialized Recipes Nutrient Rich*

Various recipes have and do call for foods especially rich in certain nutrients usually deficient in the diet. As we saw with the corn and bean combination, complementation, and also dietary supplementation, have long been a part of the human experience.

Eskimos who continue to hunt eat caribou rumen contents, which consist mostly of lichens and bacteria, on a fairly regular basis. Such a dietary adjunct, even in relatively small quantities, supplies a good amount of vitamins because of bacteria synthesis during fermentation.

*Clay, a Mineral Supplement*

Clay has until recently also been used by Eskimos. A montmorillonite clay called Umiat bentonite, primarily from a now-deserted locale, Umiat, was spoken of by local peoples who used it as "sweet" to taste and those who ascribed it therapeutic properties traveled every few years to Umiat to renew their supplies. It is established that bentonite clays are very effective absorbing agents, especially of toxic substances.

Another example of dietary supplementation is the recipe for Coquilles St.-Jacques. As served in an African restaurant in Brussels, Belgium, this dish calls for ground-up clamshells, a rich calcium source. Ground shells of various sea creatures are also eaten in West Africa, notably the Ivory Coast, while on the Prince Edward Islands in the southeast corner of Africa they are an important dietary constituent.

Throughout the world we encounter recipes for shellfish of the soft-shell variety, such as shrimp, where the entire exoskeleton is eaten, a good source of chitin as roughage.

*Plant Ash, a Mineral Adjunct*

The Hopi Indians often added plant ash or native crude salt during food preparation. The predominant whole-grain, mature maize products being high in phytate, which may interfere with absorption of some minerals, was thus wisely overcome. Thus, the porotic hyperostosis ("holes in the bones") found in skeletal remains of ancient Hopis may well have been due to a lack of iron, or to other mineral deficiencies, especially if plant ash was only recently added to the diet, and certainly when animal foods were in limited supply.

A survey of plants in Panama by Covich and Nickerson confirms that here too vitamin supplements are derived from many cultivated plants. The Chocó, who live along a large river in Panama's Darién Province, subsist mainly on upland rice and plátano *(Musa paradisiaca),* a type of plantain. In addition to these staple foods, up to fifty other useful species are cultivated in gardens. These plants are said to be vitamin rich and are of great importance in an otherwise restricted diet.

*Supplements Necessary to Maintain Health*

And so, while vitamin and mineral supplementation is an ancient theme, we must not rush to the conclusion that if a little is good, a lot is better. There is definitely a need for supplements, even for "healthy" people, but just *how much* we need, on a preventive basis, to overcome the famine within, is a matter of much controversy.

To establish standards of human nutrient requirements the RDAs, or Recommended Dietary Allowances, have been established. But as we will see, these recommendations are really only a starting point. Nevertheless we must evaluate these standards since all foods in this country which list ingredients do so with specific reference to the RDAs.

# Uses and Misuses of the RDAs

*RDAs, a Product of Emergency Planning*

As we have seen, the early religious and culturally based dietary laws were primarily aimed at prohibiting the use of adulterated and spoiled foods or maintaining cultural integrity. It wasn't until the advent of "scientific nutrition" that more formal recommendations concerning the dietary intake of specific nutrients could be made. Human nutrient requirements began to be estimated in the early 1920s, and the first nutritional standards were issued in 1935 by the Technical Committee on Nutrition of the League of Nations. This agency limited its recommendations to energy and protein needs, with the primary purpose of determining the minimal amount of food that people required so that it could be supplied in emergencies such as wars, where normal food supplies might be cut off.

With the growing threat of U.S. involvement in World War II, a Committee on Foods and Nutrition was established in 1941 in the National Academy of Sciences–National Research Council. In that same year the Food and Nutrition Board published the first Recommended Dietary Allowances, or RDAs, for various nutrients; subsequent revisions have taken place about every five years, the latest in 1979. These RDAs continue to be used as the official guidelines for practically "all nutritional enterprises in this country. They have served as the accepted yardstick for feeding the armed forces; they have unified concepts of nutritional allowances and have stimulated research to determine the requirements for the various nutrients" (FNB, January 1978).

*Standards Not Meant for Individual Needs*

How are these requirements established? The RDA for a given nutrient is determined by reviewing all the scientific evidence and defining the *mean* quantity of that nutrient that a population requires. This means that half the people eating less than this quantity might show *no* signs of deficiency, and that half of those with an intake *exceeding* the mean may show signs of deficiency. The quantity stipulated depends, of course, on how we define *requirement*—whether it is the amount that will just prevent a deficiency disease, or the amount that will cure a deficiency disease, or the quantity that will maintain an optimal saturation level of the nutrient in the body. Regardless of the definition, the initial estimate is the mean; to allow for variability among individuals, the actual RDA is set at two standard deviations above this mean, which means that 98 percent of all healthy persons in the American population will have their needs for that specific nutrient satisfied by the amount specified. Of course, this amount obviously exceeds by a huge margin the minimal nutrient requirement for some individuals in the population.

*RDAs Misused*

The RDAs were first created in response to the threat of war, in an effort to define nutrient needs for mass feeding programs, in which whole populations might need to be supplied with minimal diets. Over the years the use of the RDAs has changed, and there is now considerable confusion because they are being applied for purposes for which they were never intended. Presently the RDAs have at least three main uses: (1) as guidelines for designing diets to meet certain nutrient requirements; (2) as standards for evaluating dietary data or nutritional status; (3) as standards for use by government regulatory agencies.

*Standards Inadequate*

Obviously, since the RDAs were originally intended to be applied to groups, they are at best only a starting point for determining the adequacy of nutrient intake for an individual. Nor do the RDAs take into account the possible interactions between nutrients, or the changes that take place in these nutrients as they go through the various phases of food processing. Nutrients are not purchased as such but are incorporated into food, which must be harvested, shipped, processed, preserved, and cooked; what consumers should be concerned with is not the amount of a given nutrient in a package, but how much reaches the cells in their bodies.

Another problem with the RDAs is that they have largely focused on the micronutrients, with less emphasis on the biological action of the macronutrients. Furthermore, since the institution of the RDAs in the 1940s our foods have been undergoing significant changes, and many of the components found in foods today, particularly harmful additives, have not been addressed in the RDAs.

*Additives
Ignored*

In 1973 the Food and Drug Administration decided to incorporate the RDAs into regulations on food labeling. Known as the United States RDAs, these were based on the 1968 edition of the RDAs. This was the first time that the RDAs were officially used by regulatory agencies in prescribing nutrient intakes for members of the population, especially those receiving federal assistance. There was no provision in the FDA regulations to update these U.S. RDAs on the basis of new editions of the RDAs.

Not only are the RDAs inappropriate for measuring individual nutritional status, but we might also ask whether the focus on "dietary deficiencies" in the United States might not be failing to address the most serious nutritional problems in this country. The U.S. population may not be suffering so much from undernutrition of specific nutrients as from overnutrition or maldistribution of the macronutrients. In recent years medical and nutritional researchers both within and outside of government agencies have raised the possibility that certain dietary excesses may be associated with various disease states.

*Wrong Focus
Emphasized*

The Senate Select Committee on Nutrition and Human Needs (the McGovern Committee) recently attempted to educate the public about the dangers of such dietary imbalances by issuing its "Dietary Goals." These Dietary Goals, which are discussed in detail in Chapter 13, "A Strategy for Daily Dining," aroused considerable controversy within medical and scientific circles—partly, one suspects, because it was a legislative committee rather than a body within the medical or scientific establishment that issued these sensible dietary recommendations. The Dietary Goals remain politically charged today. Their recommendation that the amount of fat and meat in the American diet be reduced, for example, poses a threat to several large food industries, while suggestions that we also moderately reduce our intake of sugar and other refined carbohydrates, as well as alcohol, have stimulated another industrial giant to buy full-page advertisements in major American newspapers, where their version of "Sane Facts About Nutri-

*Dietary
Excesses
Emphasized by
Wise Political
Body*

tion" is little more than the Orwellian vision of *1984,* where lies become truths.

*National Health Could Improve*

The suggested changes in the national diet can be applied to *any* ethnic foods. By reducing the relative proportions of fats, protein, and alcohol; eliminating additive-containing foods; and switching to whole grains, the national health would benefit greatly, without disrupting agricultural or trade policies, if implemented gradually. Industrial panic, typical of corporate "thinking," represents fears based on executive knowledge of the inadequacy of nutrient levels in many of their products.

*Invisible Famine Serious*

To overcome the internal invisible famine *we* must select our foods differently—and by choosing wisely affect marketing decisions, which will gradually create a more wholesome national diet.

To better comprehend these dietary goals, we must first look at the nutrients in relation to the RDAs, which, having a limited but extremely important meaning, will give our specific discussion of each nutrient type greater significance.

# The Nutrients

*Forty to Fifty Known Nutrients*

Living organisms, whether animals or plants, consist of an unknown number of different organic compounds, which have been estimated at from 100,000 to possibly several million. Most of these are manufactured by the organism; however, approximately forty to fifty different known substances must be ingested in order for the organism to survive. It is these ingested chemical substances that the science of nutrition has defined as its arena of interest. A great deal of progress has been made in the past hundred years in understanding the chemistry of these substances and much of their mode of action, and in many instances even the quantities in which they must be taken.

This rather narrow definition of the science of nutrition is not completely satisfactory, because we ingest not only these nutrients, but we also ingest material which we call food. We ingest food because it is the carrier of these nutrients, but food also contains many chemicals which may be manufactured by the animals or plants themselves; or it may contain additives, either inadvertent or intentional. These chemicals may be inert, or they may have beneficial or adverse effects upon us.

*Food Symbolism Profound*

Even beyond this, food has taken on tremendous symbolic significance for the human species; with the diversity of human cultures the symbolic meaning of food has been extremely varied. Food has therefore been a very powerful psychological and social tool in man's history. No festival, no holiday, is complete without special foods for the occasion.

When talking about food, then, or nutrition, we must remember that we are not only talking about the study of the essential nutrients, but also about the vast cultural sweep of history.

*Food Not Separate from Culture*

Given these parameters, we can divide the nutrients into two large classes. The first class is referred to as the *macronutrients*. These are substances which we need in relatively large quantity. They include both the building blocks for all of the chemical machinery of the body—primarily the proteins—and the materials supplying mainly energy—the carbohydrates and fats.

*Macronutrients, Micronutrients, Defined*

The second broad category is called the *micronutrients*. These include the *vitamins*, which are organic materials found mainly in plants (except for one, vitamin $B_{12}$, which is manufactured only by microorganisms), and the *minerals*, elements which are part of the earth's crust, and which must be ingested in amounts ranging from relatively large quantities of several grams per day (calcium) down to trace amounts which are measured in parts per million or parts per billion of our diet (example: selenium). In addition, of course, we all require water for life. It is these chemical substances that we need to look at. Before doing so we must divert to an understanding of energy, the fundamental requirement.

*BULLSHIT NEGATIVE LEARNING*

# Life, Death, and Energy

All living things require energy in order to survive and to carry out their functions. Energy is necessary to maintain those processes of which we are totally unconscious but which are occurring constantly in all of us—the constant flux of chemical reactions, of electrical phenomena, of the beatings of our heart—as well as the sensations and perceptions that we receive from the external world, and the interpretation and integration of these by our central nervous system. When energy flow ceases, the organism is declared dead.

*Energy Is Life*

Many of the concepts that originated in ancient Eastern medicine, concerning energy flows as characterizing life and energy flows as being associated with disease, are not very far from the concepts of modern biochemistry and nutrition, which recognize the constant need for energy flow.

*Disease as Blocked Energy Flow*

*Death and Life*
*Defined by*
*Activity*

There is absolutely no difference in terms of compounds and molecules between the living person and the dead person; the only difference is that the live person has his molecules in active motion as a result of energy flow, whereas in the dead person these molecules no longer are associated with changes in energy state.

The exact manner in which the human organism utilizes energy derived from foodstuff is not entirely understood at the most fundamental molecular level, but it is quite well understood in terms of the energy transfers and changes in these compounds. In fact, we can even quantify the amount of energy that can be derived from the various foodstuffs which are ingested.

*Energy as Heat*

Energy availability, or energy expenditure, can be expressed in various ways. In animal organisms it is commonly expressed in terms of heat equivalents, with the unit of measure being the *kilocalorie;* when we speak of the number of calories in a given food, we are speaking of nutritional or animal calories, which should really be called kilocalories (abbreviated kcal), each of which is equal to one thousand of the calories as defined by the engineer. The reason this energy is expressed in terms of heat is that virtually all bodily energy processes are ultimately converted into heat, and it is therefore possible to measure the total energy expenditure of the organism by measuring the total amount of heat that the organism puts out. As we have seen, Lavoisier and others demonstrated that man was in certain ways similar to a burning candle, in that both of them generated heat.

How much energy can be derived from each of the major foodstuffs? The values below are those generally given for the carbohydrates, fats, and proteins as classes of compounds, and refer to the amount of energy that is available to the organism from these foodstuffs. This is not necessarily the total amount of energy that could be released if the foodstuff could be totally utilized; certain substances, particularly protein, cannot be totally degraded. Within each class of compounds specific substances may have different values, and sometimes the differences may be quite significant, a deviation of as much as 10 percent to 20 percent from the average value. The energies are as follows:

Carbohydrates = 4 kcal per gram

Fat           = 9 kcal per gram

Protein       = 4 kcal per gram

Where is the energy in the foodstuffs? The energy occurs in the chemical bonds, and it is only those chemical bonds that the organism is able to break that yield energy when broken. These are the chemical bonds between carbon atoms and between carbon and hydrogen atoms. There are other types of bonds, such as bonds between carbon and oxygen and between nitrogen and hydrogen, which are unavailable as a source of energy because animals have never developed in their evolution the capability of breaking these bonds. These substances are therefore excreted in some form and energy potentially available from such bonds cannot be utilized by the animal organism. *Energy in Chemical Bonds*

How did the energy get placed in these chemical bonds? All of the energy that the animal organism utilizes are derived from the sun, with small contributions from other parts of the universe, and largely consists of a small part of the spectrum, corresponding to the ultraviolet portion. *Sun Source of All Energy*

This ultraviolet band of energy acts upon chlorophyll, the green coloring matter of plants, which is the substance that captures the sun's energy and forms the chemical bonds of the fat, carbohydrate, and protein which are then ingested by animal organisms. *Chlorophyll as Energy Converter*

It is possible for the animal organism to reorganize and reorient some of these chemical bonds, especially to foodstuffs. For example, if excess carbohydrate is taken, this material is not burned but is converted into fat. Similarly, the body is able to manufacture certain of the building blocks of protein from chemical substances as long as sufficient nitrogen in a certain form has been supplied to the organism. *Energy Converted*

Thus the organism, although dependent in large measure upon all of the foodstuffs mentioned above for its energy, may as a result of these interconversions utilize these materials in vastly different proportions and still maintain itself in a reasonable state of health.

Let us now examine the compounds that occur within each category of foodstuffs and their respective physiological effects.

## The Macronutrients

Among the macronutrients are the foodstuffs that we must ingest to furnish the fuel for maintaining our life processes. Required in considerable amounts, these substances constitute the major part of our diet.

*Polymers*
*Composed of*
*Simpler*
*Substances*

All of the macronutrients are polymers of simpler substances; a polymer is merely a large molecule made up of repetitious chemical combinations of the same or closely related compounds. The number of simple building blocks in the polymer can vary from as few as two to the thousands and tens of thousands, and both the size and the methods of chemical linkage can have very different biochemical effects within the body.

Until recently it was thought that on ingestion these large polymers would always be degraded in the intestinal tract to their simple building blocks, and that most of these building blocks would then be reconstructed within the body in the special manner that the organism requires, and that therefore each group of polymers would have essentially the same biochemical and physiological effects. We now know this is not the case.

## The Proteins

*Proteins*
*Composed of*
*Amino Acids*

The proteins are composed of polymers derived from simple building blocks known as amino acids (A.A.'s). There are twenty-two different amino acids known to be found in animal organisms. These amino acids can be arranged in a variety of permutations and combinations with repetitions in the area of thousands or tens of thousands, so that there is a virtual infinity of different combinations. Each of these combinations has different potential physical as well as biochemical functions. The proteins constitute the machinery that drives the chemical reactions, namely, the enzymes, and also form the basis of the structural components of our bodies—the bones, tendons, and muscles.

*Eight Amino*
*Acids Cannot*
*Be Made*
*Within*

Of the twenty-two basic building blocks, the amino acids, at least eight are what are known as essential; that is, the body *cannot* manufacture them and must acquire them by ingestion. In the young child two more may be necessary, but in adulthood all the others can be manufactured within the body from non–amino acid precursors. All that is required are the precursors and enough nitrogen in the form of amino groups to manufacture these amino acids, which are then synthesized or made into necessary proteins by each individual cell, or in some cases by the liver, and discharged into the bloodstream.

*Animals and*
*Plants Supply*
*Essential A.A.'s*

Where do we get these amino acids, and how can we be certain that we have sufficient quantity? At the time that requirements were being determined for proteins and amino acids, it came to be recognzied that protein derived from animal sources has an amino-acid composition closer to that of our bodies than the amino-acid composition of the proteins from plant sources. Hence it was assumed that animal proteins were "of higher biological value," that they could satisfy the amino-acid needs of the organism more efficiently; that is, at a lower concentration, because they were a more complete protein than plant proteins. They were also considered more digestible and more easily assimilable. The early nutritionists therefore put a great deal of emphasis upon animal protein. However, as our methods for analyzing amino acids improved, and our knowledge of requirements increased, it became clear that the primary problem was that of obtaining a sufficient quantity of essential amino acids, and that it makes very little difference whether they are obtained from plant or animal sources, or even synthetic amino acids, although such synthetics would obviously be an unpalatable and expensive way to obtain our amino-acid diet. We have learned that certain plants have relatively low concentrations of certain amino acids, while other plants have a surfeit of these amino acids and are lower in others; so through complementary use of various plant sources we can obtain as satisfactory an amino-acid mixture as from animal protein.

As we saw in "The Ethnic Factor," bean protein, for example, is usually low in one of the required amino acids, methionine, but is relatively high in lysine; while the contrary is true of wheat protein, which is relatively low in lysine but realtively high in the sulfur-containing amino acids such as methionine. Therefore the combination of wheat and/or corn and beans constitutes a protein very similar to animal protein. *Wheat Plus Beans Provide All Essential A.A.'s*

Why, then, all the fuss about the need for meat protein? The problem is really one of obtaining adequate quantities of essential amino acids. In the case of animal proteins, whether from meat, eggs, milk protein, etc., the amino acids can be obtained in a relatively concentrated manner. From an ecological point of view, however, the production of this protein is accomplished with a serious energy deficit. Animal proteins must be converted by some animal from plant sources. If the plant sources are not otherwise edible and digestible by man, then these proteins constitute a net gain; that is, if the animal is allowed to graze on land that cannot produce food for man. However, when the animals are fed food that could be eaten by humans, as in the production of beef, it requires approximately eight to ten times the amount of protein derived from *Animal Protein Energy Expensive* vegetable sources to produce one part of animal protein, a serious net loss which from a biological point of view is totally unnecessary. Man in other words could live on the same food that had been fed to the cattle, with a gain in efficiency of approximately eight to ten.

*Animal Protein Associated with Fat*

Moreover, we generally do not eat protein in isolation; what we eat is the whole food. In the case of grains we should be eating the whole grain; in the case of legumes, we should and frequently do eat the whole bean, although in the case of various soy products the protein may be concentrated for us, as has been done for ages in the Orient in the making of tofu, or bean curd. In the case of animal protein, the protein is usually accompanied by animal fat. In fact, over the course of time, particularly in the case of beef, the amount of fat relative to the amount of protein has been increasing, both as a result of genetic manipulation to produce fatter animals and as a result of overfeeding of the animals to produce a very fat animal.

*Tender Beef Is Fatty*

The motives for this are partly economic, to get the greatest possible weight on the animal, but it is also partly due to our desire for increasingly tender meat. One of the factors responsible for increasing the tenderness of meat is the deposition of fat, the so-called marbleization of meat. In fact, the grading of meat is based entirely on its fat content: the higher the fat content, the higher the grade of beef! We might say that the object of the beef producers is to produce a steak that is very similar to butter, and they have gradually been accomplishing this goal, not only in terms of tenderness, but also in terms of chemical composition.

The nature of this fat is a further problem, particularly in cattle, both in their meat and in their milk products. Cattle, being ruminant animals, do not absorb their foodstuff intact; the food goes into a large pouch known as a rumen where it is attacked by microorganisms. These microorganisms break the material down completely, and this broken-down material then passes on to the digestive areas of the animal. Here the various amino acids and fatty acids are absorbed, and they are resynthesized by the animal organism. The protein that is resynthesized is quite similar to the protein of our own bodies, but the fat that is manufactured is what is know as saturated fat, which is quite different from the fat found in most seeds and plant sources. This saturated fat is laid down in large quantities in the fat depots of the animal.

The fat from plants contains a different chemical bond in specific places, known as an unsaturated bond, and most plant fats consist of greater or lesser amounts of unsaturated fats, whereas animal fat, particularly that of ruminants such as the cow, comprises almost exclusively saturated fats, both in the tissues and in the milk. The animal organism is unable to manufacture the types of unsaturated fats that are necessary for normal cell function in animal and plant organisms; in fact, the cow is probably able to manufacture or to absorb just sufficient quantities of these polyunsaturated fats to enable it to survive.

HOW MUCH PROTEIN DO WE NEED? In my practice, mainly with affluent northern Californians, people consume about 100 to 125 grams of protein daily. Back in 1881, Voit studied German workers, and recommended 118 grams of protein daily—a figure reflecting the high meat consumption of these men and the fact that they performed physical labor. We can survive on *much less* protein; as little as 25 to 40 grams daily, from vegetable foods, has been found to be adequate for healthful survival.

*Low-Protein Diet Adequate*

On the extreme side it should be noted that the Eskimos of Greenland were observed to eat about 280 grams a day, showing no signs of disease of the liver and kidney, or gout. But, such a "superabundant" amount provides no advantage; in fact, the opposite may be true, especially for rather sedentary people.

*Eskimos Eat Much Protein with Impunity*

There is increasing evidence that protein in larger quantities than required may be "toxic." This is particularly true of animal proteins, where there appears to be a relationship between high animal-protein intakes and elevation of blood cholesterol. Even more important, increased amounts of protein have been shown to lead to increased quantities of calcium being lost from the body. This calcium loss, together with the relatively low calcium intake of most American adults—indeed, many populations of the world seem to subsist on relatively low-calcium diets—may be one of the factors leading to the demineralization of bone, or osteoporosis, which is such a common phenomenon of aging in humans.

*High-Protein Diets Can Induce Calcium Loss*

People who eat very large quantities of protein must *also* consume large quantities of calcium. Meats are particularly rich in phosphorus, and a calcium/phosphorus balance of 1:1 is ideal. High-phosphorus, low-calcium diets (typically American) may contribute to osteoporosis. By eating *bones* with meat a relative balance is maintained, which explains how some people manage to eat enormous quantities of meat without inducing a state of negative balance. In "The Ethnic Factor," for exam-

*Meat Has Much Phosphorus*

ple, we saw how a Chinese dish of spareribs is prepared with vinegar, because it helps transfer tricalcium phosphate from the bones into the broth, creating a good calcium/phosphorus balance.

*Bowel Cancer Related to Fat Intake*

It is important to emphasize that the ingestion of relatively large quantities of fat, saturated or unsaturated, without adequate intake of vitamins, minerals, and cellulose, may be associated with increased incidence of cancers of the bowel. Therefore, the avoidance of an exclusively high-protein/fat diet is important.

Over the last fifty to seventy years our diet has changed very markedly. Around the turn of the century over three-quarters of the protein in our diet was vegetable protein; there has now been a complete reversal, so at present about three-quarters of our protein is consumed from animal products.

## Fats

Fats are substances that are soluble in a group of materials, including gasoline, ether, benzene, chloroform, etc., which are known as fat solvents. Any substance that will dissolve in fat solvents more readily than water is referred to as a fat, or lipid. These relatively complex substances are usually divided into two main categories, triglycerides and phospholipids.

*Fats Vary in Size*

The *triglycerides* consist of three fatty acids attached to a small three-carbon sugar known as glycerol. These fatty acids can vary in length from two carbons up to twenty or more carbons, although most are in the sixteen- to eighteen-carbon range. They can also be saturated fatty acids—that is, with all the carbons being connected by single bonds—or they can have varying degrees of unsaturated fat. For example, linoleic acid,* an eighteen-carbon fatty acid with two unsaturated bonds in critical positions, is essential for normal cell function, and is the only essential fatty substance that must be ingested.

The triglycerides are so named because they contain three fatty-acid chains, one attached to each of the three carbon atoms in glycerol. The total number of permutations and combinations of these triglycerides is enormous. These are the fats we usually ingest.

*Lecithin Mainly a Phospholipid*

The other large class of fats, known as *phospholipids,* contain two fatty-acid chains attached to two of the carbons of glycerol,

---

* Linoleic acid is found in abundance in safflower, corn, and sunflower seed oil (*not* in olive oil). Our daily requirement for this nutrient is about 3 to 5 grams, which is easily met by one tablespoonful of any of these oils.

but the third carbon, instead of having a fatty-acid chain, has a complex group of molecules containing phosphorus with an organic nitrogen base; hence the name phospholipids. These are characteristically found in materials such as lecithin, as well as in membranes and circulating within the bloodstream.

There are other types of fats associated with sugars, some associated with proteins and other moieties, as well as compounds extracted with the lipid solvents, such as cholesterol. It is only from the fatty acids and glycerol that energy can be obtained. Cholesterol does not give rise to energy, and neither do the phospholipids. Except for linoleic acid, all of the fats can be synthesized by animals and plants from simpler sources, and the usual starting point for forming these fats is excess quantities of carbohydrates. The fatty acids can also be shortened or lengthened—but generally lengthened—by the animal organism. *Cholesterol Yields No Energy*

How do we recognize which fats are saturated and which are unsaturated? In general, the longer the fatty-acid chain, the greater the tendency of fat to become solid at higher temperatures. This is one of the reasons why animal fats are usually solid at room temperature. The other factor affecting physical characteristics is unsaturation; the greater the degree of unsaturation, irrespective of chain length, the greater the tendency of that fat to become liquid at lower temperatures. Therefore most vegetable fats, which are usually high in polyunsaturated fats, are liquid. Some fatty acids are not polyunsaturated, which means having two or more double bonds; some, called monounsaturated fats, contain only one double bond, and these constitute one of the commonest sources of fat in the fat foods we consume. *Unsaturated Fats More Liquid*

Until recently it was believed that a diet relatively high in saturated fat would tend to elevate blood cholesterol, whereas a diet higher in polyunsaturated fats would lower cholesterol. However, there is great variation among individuals in how they handle the type of fat that they eat. In general, an individual with elevated blood cholesterol can reduce it by eating more polyunsaturated fats *and* a broad spectrum of other nutrients—"notably, vitamin E, vitamin C, vitamin $B_6$, other B vitamins (choline particularly), minerals (magnesium, calcium), and trace minerals together with good sources of protein (rich in methionine) . . . in any diet containing adequate amounts of polyunsaturated fats" (Williams, 1973). *Specific Vitamins and Minerals Protect Against Heart Disease*

Blood-cholesterol level is related, as a so-called risk factor in coronary disease, to the presence of a very unusual type of circulating lipid. These lipids circulate in the blood attached to protein, which helps solubilize them, and are known as *lipoproteins.* One such lipoprotein, containing a large quantity of phospholipid, is sometimes called a high-density lipoprotein. It is not significantly influenced by diet; in fact we know little about what regulates its levels or rates of synthesis. This high-density lipoprotein is an important regulator of cholesterol levels, and may be of great significance in determining the time and rate of onset of atherosclerosis.

*Hydrogenation Alters Fats*

Another complicating factor in the question of dietary fats is the influence of technology on our diet. For years people did not like to have to handle liquid fats. It is quite easy technologically to turn a polyunsaturated fat into a saturated fat by the process of hydrogenation. This has two results. One is that it changes the physical consistency, so that the material becomes a solid at room temperature, and is much easier to handle. But fats containing a double bond tend to deteriorate much more rapidly through a process known as auto-oxidation—that is, they turn rancid.

*Questionable Chemicals Added*

This can be protected against, at least in part, by the presence of antioxidants, the main natural antioxidant being vitamin E. Certain chemicals have also been found to act as antioxidants, among these BHA and BHT. These substances will indeed inhibit hydrogenated fats from turning rancid, but it has not been definitively determined whether they are truly nontoxic.

*Alteration of Fats Biologically Questionable*

A final unresolved issue has to do with the complex physical orientation of the unsaturated fat molecule. The unsaturated fat in its normal state has a certain three-dimensional configuration in space. When this substance is tampered with, either by extremes of heat or during the process of hydrogenation, this three-dimensional structure may be altered so that the carbon-hydrogen groups may be rotated at their attached double bond. Although these molecular configurations are indistinguishable chemically, it is possible that such physical transformations may have adverse biological effects. Little has been done in examining this question.

*Butter Preferred to Margarine*

For these reasons products containing hydrogenated fats are to be avoided. Butter, in this light, is preferable to margarine, which *always* contains some hydrogenated fat, no matter whether the word *natural* is emblazoned on the package. The wisest approach, though, is to avoid butter as well. It may be more natural than margarine, but it is one of the most concentrated fats in our already fat-rich diets.

## Carbohydrates

This class of nutrients provides us with about 25 to 40 percent of our calories. It is here where some of the greatest variations in dietary recommendations occur, ranging from the "no carbohydrate" approach to almost 90 percent of the total food intake.

Chemically related, the carbohydrates are subdivided by their composition into three distinct groups:

*Three Classes of Carbohydrates*

1. *Monosaccharides* (e.g., $C_6H_{12}O_6$; one sugar group in each molecule), comprising *grape sugar* (dextrose or glucose), *fruit sugar* (fructose or levulose), and *galactose* (derived from milk sugar).

2. *Disaccharides* (e.g., $C_{12}H_{22}O_{11}$; two sugar groups in each molecule), comprising *sucrose* (saccharose or cane sugar), found in the juice of many fruits and vegetables, *maltose* (malt sugar), formed from starch by enzymatic action, and *lactose* (milk sugar), found in the milk of all mammals.

3. *Polysaccharides* [e.g., $(C_6H_{10}O_5)$ X; several sugar groups], X being a variable factor, but always exceeding 10. They include *starch,* in which form nature stores most of the carbohydrates in plants; *glycogen,* which is stored as reserve carbohydrate principally in the liver and muscular tissues of animals; *dextrins,* which are formed from starch by diastase, acid, or heat; *cellulose,* principally found in wood and in the cell walls of plants; *galactans,* which occur in seeds of legumes and cereals, and in some of the algae and lichens; and the *pectins* or jellylike bodies.

By the chemical addition of a certain amount of water the second and third groups can be converted into substances of the first. This process is called *inversion* and may be produced in a number of ways.

On a sweetness scale, the sugars rank like this:

*Fructose, the Sweetest Sugar*

| | | | |
|---|---|---|---|
| Fructose | 170 | Glucose | 74 |
| Honey | 130 | Galactose | 32 |
| Sucrose | 100 | Lactose | 18 |

These figures should be memorized, because so many health-food stores are "pushing" fructose as a substitute for sucrose, without people being fully aware that it is actually much sweeter than sucrose! This fact is also important in the treatment of alcoholism, which is often a problem of carbohydrate metabolism. Fructose is given to alcoholics to lessen their craving for drink, but may cause addiction by itself.

*Diabetics Must Avoid Fructose*

Fructose, often cheaper and definitely sweeter than sucrose, is entering the food chain at great speed. "Health foods" are often sweetened with it, especially yogurt and "natural" soft drinks, but diabetics should be warned: they *must* take insulin to metabolize fructose. Sucrose, on the other hand, stimulates the production of insulin and adrenaline, two potent secretions.

*Sucrose Empty*

People who push the safety of sucrose often tell us that this sugar occurs naturally in many fruits and vegetables. This is partially true, as shown below, but fails to explain that when separated from the cane or beets sucrose by itself does *not* contain any of the vitamins and minerals found in the natural, unrefined state. It is purely "empty" calories.

## Sucrose Levels of Various Vegetables and Fruits

| Beets | 4–5% | | Apricots | 6% |
|-------|------|---|----------|-----|
| Peaches | 7% | | Potatoes | 1.5% |
| Apples | 4% | | Peas | 3% |

*Sucrose Compared to Cocaine*

Eating refined sucrose is equivalent to taking cocaine. While part of a greater complex of chemical substances when it is found in the coca leaf,* by itself cocaine is a harsh drug. Its effects are much different when taken as part of the whole leaf, being gentler in action and relatively nontoxic.

*Lactase Required to Digest Lactose*

SUCROSE AND LACTOSE INTOLERANCE    Since it was first reported in 1959, the inability of some humans to digest lactose has become fairly well known. This simple sugar, made up of glucose and galactose, comprises up to 5 percent of the total constituents of milk. People who lack the enzyme lactase cannot digest this sugar or products that contain it. In the colon the undigested lactose is fermented by bacterial enzymes into lactic acid and other acids. Carbon dioxide and hydrogen result from the fermentation, and contribute to the symptoms of lactose intolerance, namely diarrhea, abdominal pain, gas, and abdominal distention. The blood-sugar curve is either flat or may rise a bit above the fasting level. Collected stools show a low pH (5.5 or less), especially in children and infants.

---

* Cocaine is but *one* of about seventeen alkaloids found in the coca leaf.

There are definite racial differences in the ability to digest lactose, between 70 percent and 95 percent of black people in the United States showing lactase intolerance. The incidence among American Caucasians, by comparison, varies between 6 and 10 percent. Lactase deficiency, and the concomitant inability to digest milk, is also significantly prevalent among many Asian and African peoples. Familial incidence and a fairly consistent racial distribution indicate that lactose intolerance because of lactase deficiency is inherited. As an example of the racial pattern, in Uganda Baganda children and related Bantu tribes showed this insufficiency, while people with Hamitic ancestry showed higher levels of tolerance for lactose. *Racial Differences in Lactose Intolerance*

The use of fermented or cultured milk, such as yogurt or buttermilk, is a good alternative to sweet milk for lactase-deficient people. These foods are especially rich sources of calcium and protein, and are too valuable to be omitted from diets already calcium poor. The reason lactase-deficient people have *no trouble* digesting fermented dairy products is that the process of fermentation or "culturing" changes lactose to lactic acid. Thus lactase is *not* required to digest these products and indigestion is avoided with their use.

A secondary advantage of using fermented dairy products such as "lactobacillus milk" is that the microorganisms help keep the intestinal tract healthy by promoting the growth of "friendly" microbial flora. *Lactobacillus Beneficial*

Whereas the inability to tolerate lactose is very well accepted by the medical community, few physicians have learned that other disaccharides may also be a problem for certain individuals. Congenital sucrose intolerance was reported in 1960 by Weijers, et al., and clinicians should acquaint themselves with this study to better appreciate the complaints of patients who are often dismissed as cranks. *Sucrose Intolerance a Medical Problem*

A "SWEET TOOTH" IS NATURAL    The taste for sweets is natural, and indicates a physiological demand for "energy." This demand, however, should be met only by the natural sweets found primarily in fruits. We cannot improve on nature; the total fruit or raw sugarcane also contains vitamins and minerals as well as sucrose. These are hardly the empty calories of white sugar.

The following table compares sugars with honey, molasses, and maple sugar. Note particularly how nutritious blackstrap molasses is. (On one of many investigations in the Fiji Islands I tried to buy some molasses on an out island, Ovalua, but learned that all fifty-gallon drums containing this natural sweet- *Molasses Mineral Rich* ener were always bought up by Japanese fishermen. This probably indicates an appreciation of the nutritional superiority of molasses over white sugar by the seamen.)

## Sugars, Honey, and Molasses Compared*

|  | Sugars | | Honey | Molasses |  |
| --- | --- | --- | --- | --- | --- |
|  | WHITE GRANULATED | BEET OR CANE | (STRAINED OR EXTRACTED) | (THIRD EXTRACTION OR BLACKSTRAP) | Maple Sugar |
| MINERALS: | | | | | |
| Calcium | 0 | 85 | 5 | 684 | 143 |
| Phosphorus | 0 | 19 | 6 | 84 | 11 |
| Iron | 0.1 | 3.4 | 0.5 | 16.1 | 1.4 |
| Sodium | 1.0 | 30 | 5 | 96 | 14 |
| Potassium | 3.0 | 344 | 51 | 2927 | 242 |
| VITAMINS: | | | | | |
| Thiamine | 0 | 0.01 | Trace | 0.11 | — |
| Riboflavin | 0 | 0.03 | 0.04 | 0.19 | — |
| Niacin | 0 | 0.2 | 0.3 | 2.0 | — |

* Composition in mg (per 100 g or 3½ oz).
SOURCE: "Composition of Foods," Agriculture Handbook, No. 8, U.S. Department of Agriculture. Values given vary in other sources.

Excess sugar is converted by the liver into glycogen and stored in that organ and in the muscles for future use. There is up to 300 grams of glycogen stored in the body—upwards of 1,200 calories in reserve from glycogen alone, an important survival mechanism during periods of fasting or starvation.

*Sugar Implicated in Serious Disease States*

Habitual indulgence in refined sugar causes fatty degeneration of our organs, and lays the foundation for disorders such as diabetes, coronary thrombosis, and colorectal cancer (Yudkin, 1972; Cleave and Campbell, 1966; West, 1972; Cheraskin, 1970).

*Starch a "Mother Food"*

STARCH  A "mother food," starch is the most abundant food substance, next to water, in man's diet. Starch is the foundation of all diets everywhere, found in pasta, rice, corn, potatoes, and all cereals; most of the world's peoples will not be satisfied unless a certain amount is eaten as part of a meal.

Composed of many hundreds of molecules of glucose, starch is *not* soluble in water—a factor that allows rain to fall without dissolving seeds or grains. When cooked with moist heat, starch granules absorb water; they swell and burst, forming a more readily digestible carbohydrate. To be of use to us, starch must first be broken down into its elemental glucose units, in the all-important process of chewing and the action of saliva.

It is the refining, or milling, of grains that accounts for more malnutrition in the world than any other single factor. A universal food is stripped of its outer and middle seed coat and we consequently lose all the vitamin E, all the B vitamins, and all the important fiber.

FIBER   This is the indigestible material of cereal grains and *all* vegetables that is so frequently added to foods today by proponents of preventive nutrition. Fiber consists of carbohydrates or carbohydrate derivatives which are polymerized, or formed into large molecules. Chemically, the linkages by which these large molecules are formed cannot be digested by the enzymes produced by humans or most mammals. Once thought of as being inert, fiber is now shown to have extremely important physiological actions.

*Fiber Found in All Vegetables*

For one thing, fiber can be broken down at least in part by the bacteria of the gut, and the resultant substances help to accelerate the passage of materials through the large bowel, hence avoiding constipation. Even more important, fiber has the ability to imbibe and hold water, which enables it to bind many substances found in the lower part of the small and large intestines, many of which have toxic properties. These two characteristics, the ability to bind chemical substances and to imbibe water, have an important dual effect. First, the fecal bulk is increased so that the stool remains relatively large and soft and can be easily expelled, and second, these fiber products unite with many substances which, if they were to remain within the large intestine, might have adverse effects on the large intestine itself, or might be absorbed in this area and have adverse effects in other parts of the body. This latter function of fibers is still somewhat speculative, but there is at least a suggestion that certain of these substances may help lower cholesterol by binding cholesterol and bile acids and preventing the absorption and reabsorption of cholesterol, and may also play some role in binding toxic substances manufactured by the microflora that may stimulate the production of cancer of the colon. There is less controversy concerning the water-imbibing properties of fiber. Many of the diseases of Western man, such as diverticulosis, diverticulitis, hemorrhoids, etc., are due to the straining associated with constipation, which is resolved by the addition of fiber.

*Fiber Speeds Stool*

*Traditional,*
*Whole-Grain*
*Foods Healthier*

Fiber is found only in the vegetable kingdom; the principal fibers are associated with grains, secondly with nuts, and thirdly with fruits and vegetables. So once again we return to our emphasis on whole-grain products. In removing fiber from grains in the milling process, food processors thought they were removing a substance that was inert and useless, but now we find that this allegedly inert substance plays a formidable role in the maintenance of health and the prevention of disease.

Fiber is actually made up of hundreds of different compounds, depending upon which grain, vegetable, or fruit we are looking at. About 50 percent of all fiber is made up of cellulose, about 40 percent is hemicellulose, and 10 percent is composed of other compounds (lignin, pectin, tannin, gums, etc.).

*We Must*
*Double Our*
*Fiber Intake*

Americans eat about 8 to 10 grams of fiber daily, while experts in the preventive aspects of colorectal cancer recommend between 15 to 20 grams. Blood-cholesterol levels in rats have been dramatically lowered by the addition of fiber, and this should also hold in man. Interestingly, guinea pigs require 15 percent cellulose in their diets. If we accept the relationship between this animal and man in their mutual inability to manufacture vitamin C, and our consequent need for supplements, the consumption of cellulose from foods in equal "megadoses" should prove beneficial. Here is one area where the inner famine can readily be overcome, since fiber is very abundant and inexpensive, found in all vegetable foods, especially peas, peanuts with skin intact (removing peanut skins results in a 25 percent loss of fiber), sunflower seeds, peaches, pears, apples, millet, buckwheat (kasha), wheat and all grains, lentils, and others.

*Bran Not*
*Recommended*

OVERDOING A GOOD THING: PHYTATE IN BRAN    However, as with all good things the type of food we eat to get fiber can have crucial nutritional differences. We must not overdo a good thing by mixing a few grams of bran into our recipes. Why? Because bran contains *phytate,* which complexes with a broad spectrum of metals and minerals and can induce serious deficiency states! Phytate in foods such as bran can decrease calcium absorption in the gut, decrease iron availability, decrease zinc availability, and do likewise with other important trace minerals, such as manganese, copper, and magnesium (Oberleas, 1973).

Phytates are not found in all plants and so we can consume increased amounts of fiber without also taking phytates, by selecting wisely. For this reason the following list is given to my clients, as a quick reference to fiber-rich foods, with associated relative phytate levels.

## Fiber-Rich Foods and Phytate Levels

| No Phytate | Traces of Phytate Levels | Moderate Phytate | Larger Phytate Levels |
|---|---|---|---|
| Lettuce | Green Beans | Potatoes | Cereals |
| Onions | Carrots | Sweet potatoes | Nuts |
| Mushrooms | Broccoli | Artichokes | Legumes |
| Celery | Blackberries | | |
| Spinach | Strawberries | | |
| Citrus fruits | Figs | | |
| Apples | | | |
| Pineapple | | | |
| Bananas | | | |
| Prunes | | | |

Eat *more* of the fiber-rich foods to the left of the list, to balance the overindulgence in bran presently being fostered by simplistic practitioners.

# The Micronutrients

### Vitamins

The need for vitamins by each organism, in terms of quantity and variety, is different, depending primarily upon the evolutionary history of the organism. It appears that most of the need for vitamins is the result of genetic mutations. The most primitive organisms, namely bacteria and viruses, generally have no need for vitamins, since they are able to synthesize all of them themselves. In the course of evolution mutations have occurred in plants and animals, but since vitamins were generally available in the plants that animals ingested, there have usually been no adverse effects upon the animals as a result of their having these mutations. However, in the course of evolutionary change, and with certain alterations in dietary patterns, man has at times experienced very serious vitamin deficiencies. We, as a species, have encountered considerable suffering from the failure to ingest these vitamins because of our lack of knowledge of the need for them, and because during the course of evolution we had lost the capacity to manufacture these substances.

*Need for Vitamins and Minerals a Process of Evolution*

## Vitamins and Minerals: How Much Do We Need?

*Requirements Controversial*

When we discuss vitamins and minerals, we are entering an area of considerable controversy, both within the scientific community and among those who have a vested interest in selling dietary supplements. It has long been known that deficiencies of almost any of the vitamins—and now we know that the same is true of minerals—will lead to illness of some sort. Some of the illnesses are quite specific, others rather nonspecific (these are reviewed later, in the chapter "Food as Medicine"). The essential question for each individual now is, how much of these micronutrients should he or she ingest?

In recent years certain investigators, including Dr. Linus Pauling and such associates as Dr. Arthur Robinson, as well as other physicians, including the psychiatrist Dr. Carl Pfeiffer, have reported that from their clinical observations and from laboratory experiments with animals, the variability in requirements is extremely large. They state that even if only 2 percent of the people require more of a specific vitamin than is required by 98 percent of the population (the criterion for the RDAs), this percentage can constitute significant numbers, and others may be able to improve their health by taking vitamins in quantities greater than those in the Recommended Dietary Allowances as well.

*Supplements Required*

In order to obtain vitamins in quantities significantly larger than the RDAs, it is generally necessary to consume them in concentrated or medicinal form; hence a semantic argument has arisen as to whether in these large doses they are really nutrients or whether they are being utilized for their pharmacological action. The primary arguments have centered around a few vitamins, expecially vitamin C—which Dr. Pauling considers a "type of general tonic" that is particularly effective in fighting off infectious illnesses and may possibly have effects upon cancer and also protect against heart attacks—and vitamin E, which is thought to have many potential effects upon the heart, the circulation in the extremities, and to slow the aging process. The quantities advocated for these vitamins appear astronomical—from ten to one hundred times the Recommended Dietary Allowances.

*Governmental Scientists Argue Against Supplements*

Dr. Pauling and Dr. Robinson argue that each individual has an optimal vitamin level, although the vitamin levels required for optimal health have never been clearly defined and continue to be a nagging question. The proponents of the RDAs state that they do the best they can with the scientific evidence available, and that finally someone with some expertise in this area has to examine the evidence and come up with a thoughtful educated guess. Dr. Pauling and his group counteract this by saying, yes, but these guesses are mainly guesses geared toward avoiding deficiency states.

Where in the face of this argument can we make a decision? In our affluent society there is a prevailing philosophy that more is better; we must very carefully guard against this attitude when we are dealing with materials as potent as nutrients. At least two of the vitamins are toxic, vitamin A and vitamin D; in fact, vitamin D on a weight basis is one of the most toxic chemicals known to man, and yet it is an essential material for the metabolism of calcium. Hence a ten- to hundredfold increase over the RDAs of these materials would almost certainly lead to serious toxic reactions in a large majority of people.

What about taking supplementary vitamins, and in what quantities? Many people today take vitamins, explaining that they are not sure whether they can receive adequate nutrition from the highly processed foods available in our markets. It is true that with increased amounts of fat and sugar and highly milled carbohydrates—empty calories—we must become dependent upon food with higher nutritional density or we will have to either supplement our food or supplement our diets.

I have no quarrel with individuals who desire to increase their vitamin intake by taking a supplementary vitamin pill. The problem is that many people substitute this method for a careful analysis of their total nutritional and dietary habits. They think they can eat anything they want, that all they then have to do is pop a vitamin pill into their mouth. This is an erroneous and dangerous type of thinking. Vitamin supplements are *not* by themselves the key to good nutrition. They are only one class of the many chemicals that are involved in achieving a nutritional balance for the body. The main difficulty is thinking that by merely taking a pill, which is so common in our culture, all problems will be solved. The taking of a pill does not resolve problems of good nutrition, and in fact may not even resolve the problem of vitamin deficiencies, because if we are to stick with Drs. Pauling and Robinson's argument, obviously each individual would have different requirements for each of the vitamins, and to take a vitamin pill in which the proportions are already fixed would be rather nonsensical. We would be taking too much of some nutrients and inadequate quantities of others, and Pauling and Robinson would be among

*Supplements No Substitute for Nutrition*

# Vitamins and Their Uses

| Vitamin | Source | Body Parts Affected | Bodily Functions Facilitated | Deficiency Symptoms | Therapeutic Indications |
|---------|--------|---------------------|------------------------------|---------------------|-------------------------|
| **A** | | | | | |
| Fat soluble<br><br>Augmenting nutrients:<br>B-complex, choline, C, D, E, calcium, phosphorus, zinc | Green and yellow fruits and vegetables, milk, milk products, fish-liver oil<br><br>Apricots (dried):<br>1 cup = 16,000 IU<br><br>Liver (beef):<br>¼ lb = 50,000 IU<br><br>Spinach (cooked):<br>1 cup = 8,000 IU<br><br>Carrots (raw)<br>1 med. = 10,000 IU | Bones, eyes, skin, soft tissue, teeth | Body tissue reparation and maintenance (resist infection), visual purple production (necessary for night vision) | Allergies, appetite loss, blemishes, dry hair, fatigue, itching, burning eyes, loss of sense of smell, night blindness, rough dry skin, sinus trouble, soft tooth enamel, susceptibility to infections | Acne, alcoholism, allergies, arthritis, asthma, athlete's foot, bronchitis, colds, cystitis, diabetes, eczema, heart disease, hepatitis, migraine headaches, psoriasis, sinusitis, stress, tooth and gum disorders |
| **B** | | | | | |
| Water soluble<br><br>Augmenting nutrients:<br>C, E, calcium, phosphorus | Brewer's yeast, liver, whole grains | Eyes, gastrointestinal tract, hair, liver, mouth, nerves, skin | Energy, metabolism (carbohydrate, fat, protein), muscle tone maintenance (gastrointestinal tract) | Acne, anemia, constipation, cholesterol (high), digestive disturbances, fatigue, hair (dull, dry, falling), insomnia, skin (dry, rough) | Alcoholic psychosis, allergies, anemia, baldness, barbiturate overdose, cystitis, heart abnormalities, hypoglycemia, hypersensitive children, Meniere's syndrome, menstrual difficulties, migraine headaches, overweight, postoperative nausea, stress |

| $B_1$ (THIAMINE) | | | | | |
|---|---|---|---|---|---|
| Water soluble<br><br>Augmenting nutrients:<br>B-complex, $B_2$, folic acid, niacin, C, E, manganese, sulfur | Blackstrap molasses, brewer's yeast, brown rice, fish, meat, nuts, organ meats, poultry, wheat germ<br><br>Brewer's yeast:<br>2 tbsp = 3 mg<br><br>Peanuts:<br>1¼ cups = 1 mg<br><br>Sunflower seeds:<br>1 cup = 2 mg<br><br>Brazil nuts:<br>1 cup = 3 mg | Brain, ears, eyes, hair, heart, nervous system | Appetite, blood building, carbohydrate metabolism, digestion (hydrochloric acid production), energy, growth, learning capacity, muscle tone maintenance (intestines, stomach, heart) | Appetite loss, digestive disturbances, fatigue, irritability, nervousness, numbness of hands and feet, pain and noise sensitivity, pains around heart, shortness of breath | Alcoholism, anemia, congestive heart failure, constipation, diabetes, diarrhea, indigestion, nausea, mental illness, pain (alleviates), rapid heart rate, stress |
| $B_2$ (RIBOFLAVIN) | | | | | |
| Water soluble<br><br>Augmenting nutrients:<br>B-complex, $B_6$, niacin, C, phosphorus | Blackstrap molasses, nuts, organ meats, whole grains<br><br>Almonds:<br>1 cup = 1 mg<br><br>Brussels sprouts:<br>1 cup = 2 mg<br><br>Brewer's yeast:<br>3 tbsp = 1 mg<br><br>Liver (beef):<br>¼ lb = 5 mg | Eyes, hair, nails, skin, soft body tissue | Antibody and red blood cell formation, cell respiration, metabolism (carbohydrate, fat, protein) | Cataracts, corner of mouth cracks and sores, dizziness, itching burning eyes, poor digestion, retarded growth, red sore tongue | Acne, alcoholism, arthritis, athlete's foot, baldness, cataracts, diabetes, diarrhea, indigestion, stress |
| $B_6$ (PYRIDOXINE) | | | | | |
| Water soluble<br><br>Augmenting nutrients:<br>B-complex, $B_1$, $B_2$, | Blackstrap molasses, brewer's yeast, green leafy vegetables, meat, organ meats, wheat | Blood, muscles, nerves skin | Antibody formation, digestion (hydrochloric acid production), fat and | Acne, anemia, arthritis, convulsions in babies, depression, dizziness, hair loss, irritability, | Atherosclerosis, baldness, cholesterol (high), cystitis, facial oiliness, |

# Vitamins and Their Uses (Cont.)

| Vitamin | Source | Body Parts Affected | Bodily Functions Facilitated | Deficiency Symptoms | Therapeutic Indications |
|---|---|---|---|---|---|
| pantothenic acid, C, magnesium, potassium, linoleic acid, sodium | germ, whole grains, desiccated liver<br><br>Liver (beef):<br>¼ lb = 1 mg<br><br>Prunes (cooked):<br>1 cup = 2 mg<br><br>Brown rice:<br>1 cup = 2 mg<br><br>Peas:<br>1 cup = 2 mg | | protein utilization (weight control), maintains sodium/potassium balance (nerves) | learning disabilities, weakness | hypoglycemia, mental retardation, muscular disorders, nervous disorders, nausea in pregnancy, overweight, postoperative nausea, stress, sun sensitivity |
| **B₁₂ (COBALAMIN)**<br><br>Water soluble<br><br>Augmenting nutrients:<br>B-complex, B₆, choline inositol, C, potassium, sodium | Cheese, fish, milk, milk products, organ meats, cottage cheese<br><br>Liver (beef):<br>¼ lb = 90 μg<br><br>Tuna fish (canned):<br>½ lb = 5 μg<br><br>Eggs:<br>1 med. = 1 μg<br><br>Milk:<br>1 cup = 1 μg | Blood, nerves | Appetite, blood cell formation, cell longevity, healthy nervous system, metabolism (carbohydrate, fat, protein) | General weakness, nervousness, pernicious anemia, walking and speaking difficulties | Alcoholism, allergies, anemia, arthritis, bronchial asthma, bursitis, epilepsy, fatigue, hypoglycemia, insomnia, overweight, shingles, stress |

## BIOTIN
### B-COMPLEX

| | Food sources | Body parts | Functions | Deficiency symptoms | |
|---|---|---|---|---|---|
| Water soluble<br><br>Augmenting nutrients:<br>B-complex, $B_{12}$, folic acid, pantothenic acid, C, sulfur | Legumes, whole grains, organ meats<br><br>Brewer's yeast:<br>1 tbsp = 20 µg<br><br>Lentils:<br>1 cup = 25 µg<br><br>Mung bean sprouts:<br>1 cup = 200 µg<br><br>Egg yolk:<br>1 med. = 10 µg<br><br>Liver (beef):<br>¼ lb = 112 µg<br><br>Soybeans:<br>1 cup = 120 µg | Hair, muscles, skin | Cell growth, fatty-acid production, metabolism (carbohydrate, fat, protein), vitamin B utilization | Depression, dry skin, fatigue, grayish skin color, insomnia, muscular pain, poor appetite | Baldness, dermatitis, eczema, leg cramps |

## CHOLINE
### B-COMPLEX

| | Food sources | Body parts | Functions | Deficiency symptoms | |
|---|---|---|---|---|---|
| Water soluble<br><br>Augmenting nutrients:<br>A, B-complex, $B_{12}$, folic acid, inositol, linoleic acid | Brewer's yeast, fish, legumes, organ meats, soybeans, wheat germ, lecithin<br><br>Liver (beef):<br>¼ lb = 500 mg<br><br>Egg yolks:<br>1 med. = 250 mg<br><br>Peanuts (roasted w/ skin):<br>½ cup = 190 mg | Hair, kidneys, liver, thymus gland | Lecithin formation, liver and gallbladder regulation, metabolism (fats, cholesterol), nerve transmission | Bleeding stomach ulcers, growth problems, heart trouble, high blood pressure, impaired liver and kidney function, intolerance to fats | Alcoholism, atherosclerosis, baldness, constipation, cholesterol (high), dizziness, ear noises, hardening of the arteries, headaches, heart trouble, high blood pressure, hypoglycemia, insomnia |

# Vitamins and Their Uses (Cont.)

| Vitamin | Source | Body Parts Affected | Bodily Functions Facilitated | Deficiency Symptoms | Therapeutic Indications |
|---|---|---|---|---|---|
| FOLIC ACID FOLACIN B-COMPLEX Water soluble Augmenting nutrients: B-complex, B₁₂, biotin, pantothenic acid, C | Green leafy vegetables, milk, milk products, organ meats, oysters, salmon, whole grains Brewer's yeast: 1 tbsp = 200 μg Dates (dried): 1 med. = 2,500 μg Spinach (steamed): 1 cup = 448 μg Tuna fish (canned): ¼ lb = 2,250 μg | Blood, glands, liver | Appetite, body growth and reproduction, hydrochloric acid production, protein metabolism, red blood cell formation | Anemia, digestive disturbances, graying hair, growth problems | Alcoholism, anemia, atherosclerosis, baldness, diarrhea, fatigue, menstrual problems, mental illness, stomach ulcers, stress |
| INOSITOL B-COMPLEX Water soluble Augmenting nutrients: B-complex, B₁₂, choline, linoleic acid | Blackstrap molasses, citrus fruits, brewer's yeast, meat, milk, nuts, vegetables, whole grains, lecithin Oranges (fresh): 1 med. = 400 mg | Brain, hair, heart, kidneys, liver, muscles | Artery hardening retardation, cholesterol reduction, hair growth, lecithin formation, metabolism (fat and cholesterol) | Cholesterol (high), constipation, eczema, eye abnormalities, hair loss | Atherosclerosis, baldness, cholesterol (high), constipation, heart disease, overweight |

| Nutrient | Food sources | Body parts | Body functions | Deficiency symptoms | Overdose/toxicity |
|---|---|---|---|---|---|
| **NIACIN / NIACINAMIDE**<br>**B-COMPLEX**<br>Water soluble<br>Augmenting nutrients:<br>B-complex, $B_1$, $B_2$, C, phosphorus | Grapefruit:<br>1 med. = 500 mg<br>Peanuts (roasted w/ skin):<br>1 cup = 400 mg<br>Brewer's yeast, seafood, lean meats, milk products, poultry, desiccated liver<br>Rhubarb (cooked):<br>1 cup = 80 mg<br>Chicken breast (fried):<br>½ lb = 25 mg<br>Peanuts (roasted w/ skin):<br>1 cup = 40 mg | Brain, liver, nerves, skin, soft tissue, tongue | Circulation, cholesterol-level reduction, growth, hydrochloric acid production, metabolism (protein, fat), sex hormone production | Appetite loss, canker sores, depression, fatigue, halitosis, headaches, indigestion, insomnia, muscular weakness, nausea, nervous disorders, skin eruptions | Acne, baldness, diarrhea, halitosis, high blood pressure, leg cramps, migraine headaches, poor circulation, stress, tooth decay |
| **PANTOTHENIC ACID**<br>**B-COMPLEX**<br>Water soluble<br>Augmenting nutrients:<br>B-complex, $B_6$, $B_{12}$, biotin, folic acid, C | Brewer's yeast, legumes, organ meats, salmon, wheat germ, whole grains<br>Liver (beef):<br>¼ lb = 8 mg<br>Mushrooms (cooked):<br>1 cup = 82 mg<br>Elderberries (raw):<br>1 cup = 45 mg | Adrenal glands, digestive tract, nerves, skin | Antibody formation, carbohydrate, fat, protein conversion (energy), growth stimulation, vitamin utilization | Diarrhea, duodenal ulcers, eczema, hypoglycemia, intestinal disorders, kidney trouble, loss of hair, muscle cramps, premature aging, respiratory infections, restlessness, nerve problems, sore feet, vomiting | Allergies, arthritis, baldness, cystitis, digestive disorders, hypoglycemia, tooth decay, stress |

# Vitamins and Their Uses (Cont.)

| Vitamin | Source | Body Parts Affected | Bodily Functions Facilitated | Deficiency Symptoms | Therapeutic Indications |
|---|---|---|---|---|---|
| **PABA (PARA AMINOBENZOIC ACID)** | | | | | |
| Water soluble  Augmenting nutrients:  B-complex, folic acid, C | Blackstrap molasses, brewer's yeast, liver, organ meats, wheat germ | Glands, hair, intestines, skin | Blood cell formation, graying hair (color restoration), intestinal bacteria activity, protein metabolism | Constipation, depression, digestive disorders, fatigue, gray hair, headaches, irritability | Baldness, graying hair, overactive thyroid gland, parasitic diseases, rheumatic fever, stress, infertility External: burns, dark skin spots, dry skin, sunburn, wrinkles |
| **B₁₅ (PANGAMIC ACID)** | | | | | |
| Water soluble  Augmenting nutrients:  B-complex, C, E | Brewer's yeast, brown rice, meat (rare), seeds (sunflower, sesame, pumpkin), whole grains, organ meats | Glands, heart, kidneys, nerves | Cell oxidation and respiration, metabolism (protein, fat, sugar), glandular and nervous system stimulation | Heart disease, nervous and glandular disorders | Alcoholism, asthma, atherosclerosis, cholesterol (high), emphysema, heart disease, headaches, insomnia, poor circulation, premature aging, rheumatism, shortness of breath |
| **C (ASCORBIC ACID)** | | | | | |
| Water soluble  Augmenting nutrients: | Citrus fruits, cantaloupe, green peppers Broccoli (cooked): | Adrenal glands, blood, | Bone and tooth formation, collagen production, | Anemia, bleeding gums, capillary wall ruptures, bruise easily, dental | Alcoholism, allergies, atherosclerosis, arthritis, baldness, |

| | Best Natural Sources | Body Parts Affected | Bodily Functions | Deficiency Symptoms | Therapeutic For |
|---|---|---|---|---|---|
| Augmenting nutrients: All vitamins and minerals, bioflavonoids, calcium, magnesium | 1 cup = 135 mg; Oranges: 1 med. = 100 mg; Peppers (green): 1 med. = 120 mg; Grapefruit: 1 med. = 100 mg; Papaya (raw): 1 lg. = 225 mg; Strawberries: 1 cup = 90 mg | capillary walls, connective tissue (skin, ligaments, bones), gums, heart, teeth | digestion, iodine conservation, healing (burns and wounds), red blood cell formation (hemorrhaging prevention), shock and infection resistance (colds), vitamin protection (oxidation) | cavities, low infection resistance (colds), nosebleeds, poor digestion | cholesterol (high), colds, cystitis, hypoglycemia, heart disease, hepatitis, insect bites, overweight, prickly heat, sinusitis, stress, tooth decay |
| **D (CALCIFEROL)** Fat soluble Augmenting nutrients: A, choline, C, calcium, phosphorus | Egg yolks, organ meats, bone meal, sunlight; Liver (beef): ¼ lb = 40 IU; Milk: 1 cup = 100 IU; Salmon/tuna (canned): ¼ lb = 300 IU | Bones, heart, nerves, skin, teeth, thyroid gland | Calcium and phosphorus metabolism (bone formation), heart action, nervous system maintenance, normal blood clotting, skin respiration | Burning sensation (mouth and throat), diarrhea, insomnia, myopia, nervousness, poor metabolism, softening bones and teeth | Acne, alcoholism, allergies, arthritis, cystitis, eczema, psoriasis, stress |
| **E (TOCOPHEROL)** Fat soluble Augmenting nutrients: A, B-complex, B₁, inositol, C, manganese, selenium, phosphorus | Dark green vegetables, eggs, liver, organ meats, wheat germ, vegetable oils, desiccated liver; Oatmeal (cooked): 1 cup = 7 IU; Safflower oil: 1 tbsp = 20 IU | Blood vessels, heart, lungs, nerves, pituitary gland, skin | Aging retardation, anticlotting factor, blood-cholesterol reduction, blood flow to heart, capillary-wall strengthening, fertility, male potency, lung | Dry, dull, or falling hair; enlarged prostate gland; gastrointestinal disease; heart disease; impotency; miscarriages; muscular wasting; sterility | Allergies, arthritis, atherosclerosis, baldness, cholesterol (high), crossed eyes, cystitis, diabetes, heart disease (coronary thrombosis, angina pectoris, rheumatic heart |

# Vitamins and Their Uses (Cont.)

| Vitamin | Source | Body Parts Affected | Bodily Functions Facilitated | Deficiency Symptoms | Therapeutic Indications |
|---|---|---|---|---|---|
| | Vegetable oils: 1 tbsp = 12 IU<br><br>Peanuts (roasted w/ skin): 1 cup = 13 IU<br><br>Tomatoes: 2 med = 3 IU<br><br>Wheat germ oil: 1 tbsp = 40 IU | | protection (antipollution), muscle and nerve maintenance | | disease), menstrual problems, menopause, migraine headaches, myopia, overweight, phlebitis, sinusitis, stress, thrombosis, varicose veins.<br>External: burns, scars, warts, wrinkles, wounds |

GLOSSARY OF TERMINOLOGY:
U.S. RDA  U.S. Government Recommended Dietary Allowance
MDAR  Minimum Daily Adult Requirement
IU  International Units. A measure of potency for vitamins A, D, and E. In vitamin E (D-alpha) it is the tocopheryl whereby IU potency is ascertained.
mg  milligrams
μg  micrograms

This table is not intended to be used for diagnostic or prescriptive purposes. For any treatment or diagnosis of illness, please see your physician. The use of certain dietary supplements may result in allergic reactions in some individuals; consult your physician.

the first to admit that excess amounts of almost anything, including various of the so-called nontoxic vitamins, might be injurious to some people. Therefore, although people may take vitamin pills as some additional assurance, it is erroneous to consider them a general health tonic or a substitute for good nutrition.

The preceding table lists the known vitamins, their functions, foods rich in them, and their therapeutic indications. It is important to note that this table is *not intended to be used for diagnostic or prescriptive purposes.* For any treatment or diagnosis of illness it is advised that you see your physician. By sharing this chart *together with* your doctor you may be able to devise your own supplement program.

## Minerals

All that we have said about the vitamins is also true of the minerals. In general the quantities of the macrominerals which must be taken would make the pills too large to take, so the quantities that are in the mineral pills usually are infinitesimal as compared with actual requirements. In the case of the microminerals, or trace minerals, we still are in our infancy in terms of knowledge of quantities, interactions, and availability of these materials in pills as compared with food, and will look at them separately.

The following table summarizes what we know about the minerals. It is *not* intended for diagnostic or prescriptive use.

## Minerals: The Hazards of Oversupplementation

Although mineral deficiency states are widespread, even in affluent societies, an overreaction by advocates of mineral supplementation has led to the inverse phenomenon—toxicity states resulting from excessive ingestion of trace minerals.

Trace minerals are essential constituents of pathways of enzymatic action for various metabolic processes. For many of these trace minerals, however, there is a narrow range of safe dosage, and consumers of nutritional supplements may not be aware of possible toxic effects until they actually experience kidney failure.

Perhaps the best-known example of an essential mineral that is potentially lethal in high doses is lithium, a drug commonly used today in the treatment of manic-depressive disor-

# Minerals and Their Uses

| Mineral | Source | Body Parts Affected | Bodily Functions Facilitated | Deficiency Symptoms | Therapeutic Indications |
|---|---|---|---|---|---|
| CALCIUM | | | | | |
| Augmenting nutrients: A, C, D, iron, magnesium, manganese, phosphorus | Milk, cheese, molasses, yogurt, bone meal, dolomite<br><br>Almonds:<br>1 cup = 325 mg<br><br>American cheese:<br>1 slice = 200 mg<br><br>Liver (beef):<br>¼ lb = 500 mg | Blood, bones, heart, skin, soft tissue, teeth | Bone/tooth formation, blood clotting, heart rhythm, nerve tranquilization, nerve transmission, muscle growth and contraction | Heart palpitations, insomnia, muscle cramps, nervousness, arm and leg numbness, tooth decay | Arthritis, aging symptoms (backache, bone pain, finger tremors), foot/leg cramps, insomnia, menstrual cramps, menopause problems, nervousness, overweight, premenstrual tension, rheumatism |
| CHROMIUM | | | | | |
| | Brewer's yeast, clams, corn oil, whole-grain cereals | Blood, circulatory system | Blood-sugar level, glucose metabolism (energy) | Atherosclerosis, glucose intolerance in diabetics | Diabetes, hypoglycemia |
| COPPER | | | | | |
| Augmenting nutrients: cobalt, iron, zinc | Legumes, nuts, organ meats, seafood, raisins, molasses, bone meal<br><br>Brazil nuts:<br>1 cup = 4 mg<br><br>Soybeans:<br>1 cup = 2 mg | Blood, bones, circulatory system, hair, skin | Bone formation, hair and skin color, healing processes of body, hemoglobin and red blood cell formation | General weakness, impaired respiration, skin sores | Anemia, baldness |

| Mineral | Augmenting nutrients | Sources | Body parts | Function | Deficiency symptoms | Associated conditions |
|---|---|---|---|---|---|---|
| IODINE | | Seafood, kelp tablets, salt (iodized) | Hair, nails, skin, teeth, thyroid gland | Energy production, metabolism (excess fat), physical and mental development | Cold hands and feet, dry hair, irritability, nervousness, obesity | Atherosclerosis, hair problems, goiter, hypothyroidism |
| IRON | $B_{12}$, folic acid, C, calcium, cobalt, copper, phosphorus | Blackstrap molasses, eggs, fish, organ meats, poultry, wheat germ, desiccated liver<br>Liver (beef): ¼ lb = 200 mg<br>Shredded wheat: 1 biscuit = 30 mg | Blood, bones, nails, skin, teeth | Hemoglobin production, stress and disease resistance | Breathing difficulties, brittle nails, iron deficiency anemia (pale skin, fatigue), constipation | Alcoholism, anemia, colitis, menstrual problems |
| MAGNESIUM | $B_6$, C, D, calcium, phosphorus | Bran, honey, green vegetables, nuts, seafood, spinach, bone meal, kelp tablets<br>Bran flakes: 1 cup = 90 mg<br>Peanuts (roasted w/ skin): 1 cup = 420 mg<br>Tuna fish (canned): ½ lb = 150 mg | Arteries, bones, heart, muscles, nerves, teeth | Acid/alkaline balance, blood-sugar metabolism (energy), metabolism (calcium and vitamin C) | Confusion, disorientation, easily aroused anger, nervousness, rapid pulse, tremors | Alcoholism, cholesterol (high), depression, heart conditions, kidney stones, nervousness, prostate troubles, sensitivity to noise, stomach acidity, tooth decay, overweight |

*Minerals and Their Uses* (Cont.)

| Mineral | Source | Body Parts Affected | Bodily Functions Facilitated | Deficiency Symptoms | Therapeutic Indications |
|---|---|---|---|---|---|
| **MANGANESE** | Bananas, bran, celery, cereals, egg yolks, green leafy vegetables, legumes, liver, nuts, pineapples, whole grains | Brain, mammary glands, muscles, nerves | Enzyme activation, reproduction and growth, hormone production, tissue respiration, vitamin $B_1$ metabolism, vitamin E utilization | Ataxia (muscle coordination failure), dizziness, ear noises, loss of hearing | Allergies, asthma, diabetes, fatigue |
| **PHOSPHORUS** Augmenting nutrients: A, D, calcium, iron, manganese | Eggs, fish, grains, glandular meats, meat, poultry, yellow cheese  Calf liver: ¼ lb = 600 mg  Milk/yogurt: 1 cup = 230 mg  Eggs (cooked): 1 med. = 110 mg | Bones, brain, nerves, teeth | Bone/tooth formation, cell growth and repair, energy production, heart muscle contraction, kidney function, metabolism (calcium, sugar), nerve and muscle activity, vitamin utilization | Appetite loss, fatigue, irregular breathing, nervous disorders, overweight, weight loss | Arthritis, stunted growth in children, stress, tooth and gum disorders |
| **POTASSIUM** Augmenting nutrients: vitamin $B_6$, sodium | Dates, figs, peaches, tomato juice, blackstrap molasses, peanuts, raisins, seafood  Apricots (dried): 1 cup = 1,450 mg  Bananas: 1 med. = 500 mg | Blood, heart, kidneys, muscles, nerves, skin | Heartbeat, rapid growth, muscle contraction, nerve tranquilization | Acne, continuous thirst, dry skin, constipation, general weakness, insomnia, muscle damage, nervousness, slow irregular heartbeat, weak reflexes | Acne, alcoholism, allergies, burns, colic in infants, diabetes, high blood pressure, heart disease (angina pectoris, congestive heart failure, myocardial infarction) |

Flounder (baked):
¼ lb = 650 mg

Potatoes (baked):
1 med = 500 mg

Sunflower seeds:
1 cup = 900 mg

| Mineral / Augmenting nutrients | Sources | Function | Body parts | Deficiency symptoms | Conditions |
|---|---|---|---|---|---|
| **SODIUM** <br> Augmenting nutrients: vitamin D, potassium | Salt, milk, cheese, seafood | Normal cellular fluid level, proper muscle contraction | Blood, lymph system, muscles, nerves | Appetite loss, intestinal gas, muscle shrinkage, vomiting, weight loss | Dehydration, fever, heat stroke |
| **SULFUR** <br> Augmenting nutrients: B-complex, $B_1$, biotin, pantothenic acid | Bran, cheese, clams, eggs, nuts, fish, wheat germ | Collagen synthesis, body tissue formation | Hair, nails, nerves, skin | Not known | Arthritis <br> External: skin disorders (eczema, dermatitis, psoriasis) |
| **ZINC** <br> Augmenting nutrients: A (high intake), calcium, copper, phosphorus | Brewer's yeast, liver, seafood, soybeans, spinach, sunflower seeds, mushrooms | Burn and wound healing; carbohydrate digestion; prostate gland function; reproductive organ growth and development; sex organ growth and maturity; vitamin $B_1$, phosphorus, and protein metabolism | Blood, heart, prostate gland | Delayed sexual maturity, fatigue, loss of taste, poor appetite, prolonged wound healing, retarded growth, sterility | Alcoholism, atherosclerosis, baldness, cirrhosis, diabetes, internal and external wound and injury healing, high cholesterol (eliminates deposits), infertility |

ders. In Roman times people with bipolar depressive disorders bathed in pools rich in lithium, long before the current concept of "orthomolecular" treatment was developed. Today psychiatrists must continuously monitor serum lithium levels to prevent a toxic overload and an electrolyte imbalance.

*Even Calcium Can Be Toxic*

Calcium, which is perhaps the most abundant mineral in the human body, also poses problems when too much is taken. This essential constituent of bone, cartilage, teeth, blood, and nerve cells is delicately balanced with other ionic complexes that neutralize its electrical valency. The calcium-magnesium complexes are also essential constituents of enzymatic pathways, and they must be taken together. If one of these minerals is used alone, it will induce different physiological effects than when the two are used in combination. Magnesium oxide, for example, is often prescribed independently for constipation, but when combined with calcium it does not promote bowel evacuation. An overdose of calcium supplements taken over a prolonged period of time may result in a malabsorption syndrome, known in the medical parlance as *hypercalcemia,* which leads to hyperossification and connective tissue disorders such as rheumatoid arthritis. Experimental research has revealed that calcium deposits may be dissolved through topical application of magnesium-based intradermal salves. Calcium, as it occurs in certain whole foods, such as dairy products, is more readily assimilable than it is in isolation as a pure supplement; this is why we recommend eating foods rich in calcium rather than ingesting this nutrient in tablet form.

*Toxic Metals May Coexist with Some Trace Minerals*

Just as calcium by itself can be toxic, so can other minerals. Although minute quantities of certain elements such as chromium and molybdenum are valuable and essential constituents of a nutritious diet, the user of self-prescribed supplements is often unaware that excessive ingestion can produce toxicity. Trace-mineral manufacturers are currently capitalizing on the public interest in the alleged benefits of trace minerals such as germanium and titanium, which have not yet been scientifically demonstrated to be essential. The sources of these minerals may be organically bound yeast, high-mineral kelp, or the salts from ancient seabeds. While these sources may have a high content of such essential minerals as selenium, chromium, and manganese, assays may also reveal high contents of lead, cadmium, mercury, and arsenic. The labeling requirements as mandated by the Federal Trade Commission and the Food and Drug Administration do not stipulate that these toxic minerals must be mentioned. Although arsenic is widely known as a highly carcinogenic toxin, it is also an essential mineral, at exceedingly low levels.

MOVING UP THE PERIODIC TABLE    We are now in danger of climbing up the periodic table, with each new "discovery" for the nutritional value of these little-known elements representing a new phase in potential nutritional iatrogenesis. Now that manganese and molybdenum are household words we have moved on to boron, silicon, rubidium, vanadium, titanium, and germanium. The future portends that we may soon witness a recommended nutritional use for the radioactive elements such as radium, berkellium, einsteinium, and the most carcinogenic element known to man, plutonium!

*Commercial Pressures Bias Scientific Reason*

SELENIUM    Marco Polo in his journeys noted that horses' hooves fell off when the animals grazed on plants from certain soils—soils which we now know were overly rich in selenium. However, in *safe* dosage this trace mineral may be one of our more important allies.

Although the toxicity of selenium was established long ago, it was not recognized as an essential dietary element before 1957. Selenium is not distributed evenly in agricultural land, and consequently many of our foods are grown in selenium-deficient soils; the incidence of arteriosclerotic and hypertensive heart disease in these areas is three times greater than among people who live in selenium-rich areas. Epidemiologic studies have also shown that mortality from breast and colon cancer is *lower* in areas of the U.S. where grains and other crops have high contents of selenium (Shamberger, 1969).

*Selenium Has Low Degree of Safety*

Many experiments demonstrate that selenium protects people against environmental carcinogens that may also damage chromosomes. Among the many biological functions of selenium are the normalization of blood pressure and the reduction of platelet aggregation. Selenium is also necessary in the prevention of liver necrosis and muscular dystrophy owing to nutritional deficiencies. Muscular dystrophy, incidentally, is associated with vitamin E deficiency states as well as selenium deficiency; in fact, vitamin E and selenium share many common functions and may occasionally substitute for each other in certain enzymatic pathways, by stimulating the immune system.

Since selenium is not essential for the growth of grains, fertilizers that are added to the soil usually do not contain selenium. The problem is aggravated by the fact that sulfates, which are present in artificial fertilizers, block the uptake of selenium in plants. In New Zealand, where soils are deficient in selenium, dietary supplementation of feed has helped the livestock industries.

*Selenium Forces Excretion of Toxic Elements*

Perhaps the greatest benefit of selenium lies in its ability to facilitate the excretion of mercury, cadmium, and other heavy metals. Cadmium, a ubiquitous toxic element which is prevalent in industrialized areas, is partially neutralized by selenium. Cadmium has been implicated as a contributing factor toward high blood pressure as well as certain forms of cancer.

The use of organic fertilizers made from sewage sludge often results in unsafe cadmium levels in produce. Milorganite is such a substance, and is made from sewage from the city of Milwaukee. Cadmium accumulates in the soil as well as in the animal body, so problems increase exponentially with time. Farm products that absorb high amounts of cadmium from the soil include leafy vegetables, potatoes, and wheat. Cadmium levels are also high in drinking water that has once contained sludge. A prolonged intake of excessive cadmium may lead to slow, subacute renal tubular damage causing hypertension. Further, a team of researchers at the Cleveland Clinic, led by Raymond Shamberger, Ph.D., reviewed the literature of twenty-five countries and found a significant positive correlation between cadmium levels and the incidence of coronary heart disease. Cadmium and selenium are known to compete for the same sulfhydryl dining sites.

Another elemental antagonist to selenium is the toxin arsenic, which is a major source of tumor growth in experimental animals. In a number of cancer experiments performed with rats, in which carcinogens such as arsenic were introduced into their diets, the incidence of tumors was reduced by selenium supplementation. Although dietary supplements of selenium may not prove to be effective in cases of advanced cancer, its role has been established as protection against the risk of developing cancer.

In addition to its role as an anticancer agent, selenium also enhances immune response and has a therapeutic effect in cases of rheumatoid and osteoarthritis. Selenium may also protect against smog, industrial pollution, cigarette smoking, and excessive radiation generated by microwave ovens and TV transmitters. As an essential component of the enzyme *glutathione peroxidase,* selenium has been shown to mediate the toxicity of ionizing radiation.

*Selenium Found in Common Foods*

One prominent sign of selenium deficiency is impaired sexual functioning in the male, since normal sperm cells contain high concentrations of selenium. The highest concentrations of this trace mineral are present in the kidney, liver, and pancreas. Among the dietary sources of selenium, particularly high concentrations are found in torula yeast. For those people who are allergic to yeast, many forms of kelp have high levels of selenium (e.g., *Macrocystis merifera*). Other foods rich in selenium include mushrooms, asparagus, garlic, and whole grains. If grown in seleniferous soils most garden vegetables, especially cabbage and potato peels, take up significant amounts.

Although selenium is recognized for its ability to neutralize the effects of free radicals (which may combine to form carcinogens in the bowel), it is important to remember that this trace mineral is toxic in high doses. The therapeutic margin is very narrow, involving millionths of a gram. At a recent conference for physicians a lecturer supporting the use of selenium urged his colleagues to give their patients a minimum daily dose of 300 μg! Since selenium is highly fat soluble,* there is a great danger of toxicity in people who take unsafe levels over a period of time. We recommend a maximum of 50 μg/day in supplementary form.

In man the symptoms of selenium poisoning include loss of hair and nails, dizziness, fatigue, and dermatitis. Such symptoms can be eliminated when patients are placed on a selenium-free diet. Classic cases of acute poisoning from eating selenium-rich plants involve a large tree from Central and South America known as "monkey's coconut" *(Lecythis ollaria)*. Strangers to Brazil and Venezuela sometimes inadvertently eat these toxic nuts, or ignore the warnings of local people who tell them that they will cause hair loss, diarrhea, and dizziness. *Loss of Hair Caused by Excess of This Trace Mineral*

If any of these symptoms occur, check the label on your multivitamin/mineral supplement and discontinue usage if it contains *any* selenium. Of course, with such symptoms any selenium supplements should be discontinued, but when "buried" in a multivitamin/mineral formula its dosage must be added on to any separate supplementation *and* food sources.

## Other Supplements

Amino acids and glandular extracts are being used today in alarming doses, for self-medicated complaints. This can be very dangerous for reasons soon to be shown. Before examining the current spectrum of supplements being sold "over the counter," we must see the context in which they are presented *Supplements Replace Drugs*

* Nutrients that are fat soluble are stored in our fat tissue and accumulate through time as more are taken in.

to the physician, in which the drug detail man is now being replaced by the supplement detailers, and "holistic" physicians are being brainwashed into exceeding the demonstrably safe dosage levels.

In order for a physician to renew his license to practice medicine, he must earn a minimum number of continuing medical education credits. Postgraduate instruction is often sponsored by medical specialty societies and held in convention centers, where there is an exhibit area filled with drug and "supplement" detail men, who talk to the doctors and sell them their wares.

*Supplements*
*Big Business*

The exhibitors do not like to approach the doctors while they are busy in their offices and preoccupied with the health of their patients. But when on "vacation" at an educational colloquium, they're more at ease. Besides, the detail men can show the doctor how to have a profitable business on the side. By establishing a holistic dispensary, staffed by paraprofessionals selling nutritional supplements and herbs at a markup ranging from 50 to 200 percent, added income is assured in the form of a sort of surcharge to the normal fee structure. The physicians are actually eliminating the pharmacist and at times the middleman, by eliminating the distributor in between.

This is why physicians often like to mix education with business and pleasure when attending these seminars. If the lectures become too technical and dry, they are eager to flood out to the exhibit floor where the salesmen hawk their wares, competing for a single sale, which could translate into a steady stream of orders.

*Some Holistic*
*Clinics*
*Deceptive*

The new "holistic clinic" is set up like the modern shopping center with its medico-dental building. Conveniently integrated into this "holistic general store" is a dispensary for vitamins, minerals, and hormones. After hearing a pep talk by a physician or chiropractor, the patient is eager to obtain relief as soon as possible and prefers to buy the drugs in the same building. It also seems much safer to get everything from the same source. Technically, only physicians are licensed to dispense medical advice, even concerning nutritional supplements. But these supplements are not subject to the same Drug Enforcement Administration codes as narcotics and minor tranquilizers; once the first prescription is given, the patient doesn't have to come back to the doctor for a refill.

*Supplements*
*Second to Foods*

While attending a medical conference recently, I surveyed the exhibitors' offerings and was overwhelmed by the variety of complexes and combinations of substances, which often made little sense. While vitamins and minerals have been supplemented since antiquity, these newer offerings, separated out from foods, are by no means a safe road to the future. In years to come we may see disorders, not yet documented, arising from overuse of these self-administered supplements. There may be a latency phenomenon in the use of certain supplements, and foods must remain our primary source of these substances, with only *minor* supplementation.

Further details regarding the use of *amino acids* (such as tryptophan for insomnia, glutamine for alcoholism) and *glandulars* as therapeutic supplements are explained in Chapter 10, "Food as Medicine." At this juncture we might pause to consider the unknown effects of interactions *between* nutrients, as exemplified by known interactions between nutrients and drugs.

# Interactions: A Further Complication

### Drug-Nutrient Interactions

We now know that we must avoid taking antacids when we are also taking tetracyclines, because of the interaction between these drugs, which decreases tetracycline's effectiveness. Similarly, we know of *some* interactions between nutrients.

But one of the difficulties in establishing nutrient requirements is that we know very little about all nutrient-nutrient interactions; one nutrient may interact with another, either suppressing or augmenting its action, but we know very little about when and how such interactions occur. Even more important is the interaction between drugs and nutrients, a problem with which our drug-taking society must become increasingly concerned.

Although many nutritionists had discussed drug-nutrient interactions, there was little research in this area until the widespread introduction of the birth control pill, and the observation that birth control pills led to marked changes in blood levels of certain of the vitamins and minerals. The question immediately arose whether these changes affected the health of the individual, or whether they were purely incidental. To date there is no clear-cut answer. In the case of trace minerals, at least, it appears that the changes are due not so much to changes in the metabolism of the trace minerals themselves, but rather to alterations in the transport proteins that carry these minerals

*Birth Control Pill Increases Need for Vitamin $B_6$*

in the bloodstream. These transport-protein levels change as a result of the action of hormones, rather than as a result of metabolic change.

In the case of some of the vitamins, particularly vitamin $B_6$ or pyridoxine, the effect of birth control pills has not yet been settled. A fairly high percentage of women taking birth control pills appear to have an increased requirement for this vitamin. The blood levels of $B_6$ in women on birth control pills tends to drop, and in some people quite large doses are necessary to restore the blood levels to normal. A deficiency of vitamin $B_6$ seems to lead to a feeling of depression, a very common complaint, at least initially, among many women on the pill. Clinical studies indicate that when relatively large quantities of vitamin $B_6$ are given to restore the blood level, the depression tends to lift.

In other instances the interaction is of a different sort. For example, the absorption of iron from the intestinal tract is enhanced by the presence of vitamin C, whether the vitamin C is from foods or pills. In such cases vitamin C acts to increase the blood stores of iron.

The following table shows a few of the areas where drug and nutrient interactions may play an important role—a possibility that is too frequently overlooked by the physician when prescribing drugs.

The skeptical physician should be encouraged when reviewing the above table of drug-nutrient interactions; the information provided is from the medical literature, mainly refereed journals. Anecdotal information has *not* been included for the sake of influencing practitioners in this profoundly neglected area. A complete survey is represented in *Drug-Induced Nutritional Deficiencies* by Daphne Roe, M.D. (1976), where the reader is referred for more detailed information. The following chart is from Dr. Roe's book, and should not be overlooked during *any* clinical interchange. Adverse drug reactions can mimic serious complaints but be easily offset by proper nutritional supplementation, possibly saving patient and healer from serious misdiagnosis and erroneous treatment.

## Smoking-Nutrient Interactions

In recent years it has been repeatedly demonstrated that smoking is one of the most serious health hazards to which modern man exposes himself. Smoking has been implicated in all sorts of disease, the best known including lung cancer,

# 50 Commonly Prescribed Drugs and the Nutrients They Affect

| Drug Trade Name | Major Indication(s) for Use | Major Side Effects | Nutrient(s) Affected |
|---|---|---|---|
| Achromycin | Gram negative and gram positive micro-organisms | G.I. systemic irritation<br>Skin rash<br>Kidney: rise in BUN<br>Teeth stained | Reduces absorption of calcium, magnesium, and iron |
| Aldactazide | Hypertension<br>Congestive heart failure<br>Edema | Drowsiness<br>Lethargy<br>Mental confusion<br>G.I. irritation<br>Menstrual irregularity<br>Headache | Reduced potassium excretion |
| Aldactone | Hypertension<br>Congestive heart failure<br>Edema | Drowsiness<br>Lethargy<br>Mental confusion<br>G.I. irritation<br>Menstrual irregularity<br>Headache | Reduced potassium excretion |
| Apresoline | Hypertension | Headache<br>Palpitations | Vitamin $B_6$ depletion |
| Aspirin | Minor pain | G.I. irritation | Thiamine and vitamin C deficiency |
| Atromid-S | Cholesterol control | Nausea<br>Vomiting<br>Loose stools<br>Abdominal distress | Reduction in circulating vitamin K levels |
| Azo Gantanol | Antibacterial<br>Gram negative and gram positive urinary tract infection | Headache<br>Nausea<br>Vomiting<br>Skin rash | Folic acid deficiency |
| Bentyl with Phenobarbital | Functional G.I. disorders | Dry mouth<br>Fatigue<br>Dizziness | Accelerated vitamin K metabolism |
| Betapar | Endocrine and rheumatic disorders<br>Collagen and dermatologic disease<br>Hematologic and neoplastic disorders | Fluid retention<br>Muscle weakness<br>G.I. hemorrhage<br>Convulsions | Increased $B_6$ requirement<br>Increased vitamin C excretion<br>Zinc, potassium deficiency |
| Brevicon | Oral contraception | Thrombophlebitis<br>Pulmonary embolism<br>Cerebral thrombosis<br>Nausea, vomiting<br>Migraine<br>Rash<br>Mental depression | Vitamin $B_6$ and C depletion |

## 50 Commonly Prescribed Drugs and the Nutrients They Affect (Cont.)

| Drug Trade Name | Major Indication(s) for Use | Major Side Effects | Nutrient(s) Affected |
|---|---|---|---|
| Bronkotabs and Elixir | Bronchial asthma<br>Bronchitis<br>Emphysema | Nervousness<br>Restlessness<br>Sleeplessness | Accelerated vitamin K metabolism |
| Butazolidin | Rheumatoid and osteoarthritis<br>Spondylitis | Edema<br>G.I. distress<br>Rash<br>Confusion<br>Vertigo | Folic acid deficiency |
| Cantil with Phenobarbital | Lower G.I. distress<br>Diarrhea<br>Abdominal pain<br>Cramping<br>Irritable colon | Dry mouth<br>Blurred vision | Accelerated vitamin K metabolism |
| Chardonna | Nervous indigestion<br>Gastritis<br>Nausea<br>Vomiting<br>Spastic colon<br>Flatulence | Dry mouth<br>Blurred vision<br>Vertigo<br>Tachycardia | Accelerated vitamin K metabolism |
| Colbenemid | Chronic gouty arthritis | Headache<br>G.I. distress<br>Urinary frequency<br>Dizziness | Decreased absorption of lactase, fat, sodium, potassium, and $B_{12}$ |
| Colchicine | Chronic gouty arthritis | Headache<br>G.I. distress<br>Urinary frequency<br>Dizziness | Decreased absorption of lactase, fat, sodium, potassium, and $B_{12}$ |
| Cortisone tablets and suspension | Adrenocortical deficiency<br>Allergic states<br>Rheumatoid arthritis<br>Dermatoses | Hirsutism and supraclavicular fat pads | Vitamin $B_6$ deficiency<br>Accelerated vitamin D metabolism<br>Zinc, potassium, and vitamin C deficiency |
| Cortisporin | Burns, wounds<br>Skin grafts<br>Otitis externa<br>Eczema | Systemic intolerance | Reduced lactase levels<br>Vitamin K, $B_{12}$, and folic acid deficiency |
| Demulen | Oral contraception | Thrombophlebitis<br>Pulmonary embolism<br>Cerebral thrombosis<br>Hemorrhage<br>Myocardial infarction<br>Gallbladder disease | Vitamin $B_6$ and C depletion |

## 50 Commonly Prescribed Drugs and the Nutrients They Affect (Cont.)

| Drug Trade Name | Major Indication(s) for Use | Major Side Effects | Nutrient(s) Affected |
|---|---|---|---|
| Diethylstilbestrol | Menopause<br>Senile vaginitis | Nausea<br>Vomiting<br>Vertigo<br>Anxiety<br>Thirst<br>Rashes | Vitamin $B_6$ depletion |
| Diupres | Hypertension | Nausea<br>Vomiting<br>Diarrhea<br>Dizziness<br>Vertigo | Increased magnesium and potassium excretion |
| Diuril | Hypertension | Nausea<br>Vomiting<br>Diarrhea<br>Dizziness | Increased potassium and magnesium excretion |
| Doriden | Insomnia | Skin rash | Folic acid deficiency |
| Enovid | Oral contraception | Thrombophlebitis<br>Cerebral thrombosis<br>Gallbladder disease | Vitamin $B_6$ and C depletion |
| Gantanol | Urinary tract, soft tissue, and respiratory infections | Headache<br>Nausea<br>Vomiting<br>Urticaria<br>Diarrhea<br>Hepatitis | Folic acid deficiency |
| Hydrotension Plus | Hypertension | Headache<br>Palpitations | Vitamin $B_6$ depletion |
| Indocin | Rheumatoid arthritis<br>Spondylitis<br>Degenerative joint disease of the hip<br>Gout | G.I. bleeding<br>Headache<br>Dizziness<br>Anorexia<br>Edema<br>Skin rash | Thiamine and vitamin C depletion |
| Isordil with Phenobarbital | Angina pectoris | Increased intraocular pressure | Accelerated vitamin K metabolism |
| Lidosporin | Infection pain and itching associated with otitis and furunculosis | Overgrowth of non-susceptible organisms | Malabsorption of vitamins $B_{12}$, K, and folic acid |
| Lo-Ovral | Oral contraception | Thrombophlebitis<br>Pulmonary embolism<br>Cerebral thrombosis | Vitamin $B_6$ depletion |

## 50 Commonly Prescribed Drugs and the Nutrients They Affect (Cont.)

| Drug Trade Name | Major Indication(s) for Use | Major Side Effects | Nutrient(s) Affected |
|---|---|---|---|
| Mycifradin | Enterocolitis and diarrhea | Nausea<br>Diarrhea | Reduced lactase levels<br>Vitamin K deficiency<br>Malabsorption of vitamin $B_{12}$ and folic acid |
| Mycolog | Cutaneous candidiasis<br>Infantile eczema | Localized atrophy | Reduced lactase levels<br>Vitamin K deficiency<br>Malabsorption of vitamin $B_{12}$ and folic acid |
| Neo-Cortef | Contact and allergic dermatitis | Miliaria<br>Folliculitis | Reduced lactase levels<br>Vitamin K deficiency<br>Malabsorption of vitamin $B_{12}$ and folic acid |
| Neomycin | Suppression of intestinal bacteria<br>Diarrhea | Nausea<br>Vomiting<br>Nephrotoxicity | Reduced lactase levels<br>Vitamin K deficiency<br>Malabsorption of vitamin $B_{12}$ and folic acid |
| Neosporin | Pseudomonas Staphylococcus bacteria | Overgrowth of non-susceptible organisms | Reduced lactase levels<br>Vitamin K deficiency<br>Malabsorption of vitamin $B_{12}$ and folic acid |
| Norinyl | Oral contraception<br>Hypermenorrhea | Thrombophlebitis<br>Pulmonary embolism<br>Edema<br>G.I. upset | Vitamin $B_6$ and C depletion |
| Orasone | Rheumatoid arthritis<br>Joint pain<br>Stiffness<br>Swelling and tenderness | Exaggerated hormonal effects | Increased vitamin $B_6$ requirement<br>Increase vitamin C excretion<br>Zinc and potassium deficiency |
| Os-Cal-Mone | Osteoporosis | Uterine bleeding<br>Mastodynia | Vitamin $B_6$ depletion |
| Phazyme | G.I. disturbance<br>Aerophagia<br>Dyspepsia<br>Diverticulitis<br>Spastic colitis | None | Accelerated vitamin K metabolism |
| Polysporin | Gram negative and gram positive microorganisms | Overgrowth of non-susceptible organisms including fungi | Malabsorption of vitamins $B_{12}$, K, and folic acid |
| Prednisone | Rheumatoid arthritis<br>Joint pain<br>Stiffness<br>Swelling and tenderness | Exaggerated hormonal effects | Increased vitamin $B_6$ requirement<br>Increased vitamin C excretion<br>Zinc and potassium deficiency |

## 50 Commonly Prescribed Drugs and the Nutrients They Affect (Cont.)

| Drug Trade Name | Major Indication(s) for Use | Major Side Effects | Nutrient(s) Affected |
|---|---|---|---|
| Premarin | Menopausal syndrome<br>Senile vaginitis<br>Pruritus vulvae | Uterine bleeding<br>Loss of libido | Folic acid deficiency<br>Reduced calcium excretion |
| Pro-Banthine | Peptic ulcer<br>Hypertrophic gastritis<br>Pancreatitis<br>Diverticulitis<br>Bladder spasm | Dry mouth<br>Blurry vision<br>Urinary retention | Accelerated vitamin K metabolism |
| Probital | Functional G.I. disorders | Dry mouth<br>Blurry vision<br>Urinary retention | Accelerated vitamin K metabolism |
| Ser-Ap-Es | Hypertension | Increased gastric secretion<br>Angina-like syndrome<br>Depression<br>Deafness | Vitamin $B_6$ depletion |
| Sterazolidin | Anti-arthritic<br>Anti-inflammatory | Edema<br>G.I. upset | Increased vitamin $B_6$ requirement<br>Increased vitamin C excretion<br>Folic acid, zinc, and potassium deficiency |
| Sumycin | Gram negative and gram positive microorganisms | G.I. upset<br>Anorexia<br>Nausea<br>Vomiting<br>Diarrhea<br>Dermatitis | Reduced absorption of calcium, magnesium, and iron |
| Tetracyn | Gram negative and gram positive microorganisms | G.I. upset<br>Anorexia<br>Nausea<br>Vomiting<br>Diarrhea<br>Dermatitis | Reduced absorption of calcium, magnesium, and iron |

From "Index of Nutritional Abnormalities Induced by 50 Commonly Prescribed Drugs," IMA Publications Division, Inter-Marketing Associates, Inc., La Jolla, California (1978).

## Symptoms Associated with Drug-Induced Malnutrition

| Symptom | Deficit or Condition |
| --- | --- |
| Weight loss | Protein-calorie deficit |
| Growth retardation (children) | "        "        " |
| Diarrhea | Malabsorption |
| Dermatitis of face and scalp, "burning" feet, and depression | Vitamin $B_6$ |
| Sore tongue, weakness, breathlessness | Folate |
| Dermatitis (light exposed areas), diarrhea, and confusion | Niacin |
| Bone pain, difficulty in walking; muscle (adults) weakness | Vitamin D |
| Thickening of wrists, progressive limb deformity, muscle weakness (children) | "        " |
| Bleeding gums, bruising, rectal bleeding, bleeding after injury or surgery | Vitamin K |

FROM Roe, 1976.

heart disease, impairment in the development of the fetus, and difficulties at birth and in the subsequent development of the infant. Smokers likely have increased needs for vitamin C, vitamin $B_{12}$, and vitamin $B_6$, but little research has been done in this area. In any case, the solution is very simple—namely, not to smoke. Little further comment is therefore indicated.

*Drug Effects Go Up in Smoke*    For those who must have facts, however, the following may provide the needed stimulus to quit tobacco. For one, smoking definitely interacts with a number of drugs, speeding up the process by which the body uses and eliminates them. Smokers taking any of the following drugs may need different doses or may have to take them more frequently. The drugs include theophylline, a bronchodilator used for treating asthma or bronchitis; pentazocine, a pain reliever; imipramine, an antidepressant; glutethimide, a sedative; furosemide, a diuretic; and propanolol, a beta blocker. Persons taking any of these medications must discuss their smoking with their physician.

*Blood Clots Faster in Smokers*    Other effects of smoking are equally important from a therapeutic viewpoint. For example, white blood cell counts are elevated in smokers, even when they are not suffering from an infection; the heavier the smoking, the higher the count.

Also, the blood of smokers clots faster than that of nonsmokers, a critical problem in our age when coronary heart disease is epidemic.

From a nutritional point of view it has been known for over forty years that smoking impairs protein metabolism and increases the amount of cholesterol in the blood. Bone mineral loss experienced by smokers may be related to the loss of vitamin C, and toxic trace metals in smoke may accumulate in the body. Cadmium, lead, arsenic, and radioactive polonium, present in tobacco leaves, are good reasons unto themselves for avoiding that deadly puff.

*Cholesterol Levels Increased; Nutrients Lost, Toxins Gained*

## Nutrient-Nutrient Interactions

What knowledge there is about the synergistic effects between nutrients is all positive. Little research seeking possible harmful effects has been undertaken, but this does not preclude the possibility that such untoward effects may occur.

On the positive side, we know that vitamin E prevents the oxidation of vitamins A and C, maintaining the integrity of these substances and keeping them from breaking down to combine with other elements. Riboflavin activates vitamin $B_6$ in its effects of converting tryptophan into niacin. Riboflavin is also part of the cycle in which folic acid is converted to its coenzymes and it also assists the bodily utilization of vitamin $B_{12}$, niacin, and vitamin C. Iron and vitamin $B_6$ help us to assimilate vitamin $B_{12}$, while vitamin A is more efficient when combined with the B-complex, choline, and vitamins C, D, and E. Calcium must *not* be taken by itself but in conjunction with phosphorus, in the recommended 1:1 ratio.

*Nutrients Interact*

These nutrient interactions serve to show that supplements must be carefully formulated if we are to gain advantages without laying the groundwork for nutrient-iatrogenic disorders.

For the average healthy client I recommend the following formula, which was developed by Dr. Roger Williams. It contains sufficient quantities of nutrients to offer genuine health benefits, but is *not* composed of megadoses that turn our urine yellow and stress our kidneys.

## A Note About Shopping for Supplements

Buy the established brands. I have visited the factories where "our-own-label" type preparations are composed and am impressed with the *lack* of quality control. The best assurance

*Quality Supplements Best*

## Dr. Roger Williams's Vitamin/Mineral Formulation

| | | |
|---|---|---|
| **VITAMINS:** | | |
| Vitamin A | 7,500 | units |
| Vitamin D | 400 | units |
| Vitamin E | 40 | units |
| Vitamin K (Menedione) | 2 | mg |
| Ascorbic acid | 250 | mg |
| Thiamine | 2 | mg |
| Riboflavin | 2 | mg |
| Vitamin $B_6$ | 3 | mg |
| Vitamin $B_{12}$ | 9 | $\mu g$ |
| Niacinamide | 20 | mg |
| Pantothenic acid | 15 | mg |
| Biotin | 0.3 | mg |
| Folic acid | 0.4 | mg |
| Choline | 250 | mg |
| Inositol | 250 | mg |
| P-aminobenzoic acid | 30 | mg |
| Rutin | 200 | mg |
| **MINERALS:** | | |
| Calcium | 250 | mg |
| Phosphate | 750 | mg* |
| Magnesium | 200 | mg |
| Iron | 15 | mg |
| Zinc | 15 | mg |
| Copper | 2 | mg |
| Iodine | 0.15 | mg |
| Manganese | 5 | mg |
| Molybdenum | 0.1 | mg |
| Chromium | 1.0 | mg |
| Selenium | 0.02 | mg |
| Cobalt | 0.1 | mg |

* Equivalent to 250 mg phosphorus

that you are receiving the doses stated on the label and that the formulas have been carefully manufactured is to buy quality. Avoid those health-food stores which sell "their-own-label" supplements. It is likely that they also offer a slew of other inferior products, many filled with sugar, artificial colors, artificial flavors, hydrogenated oils, and a sea of additives. These were the contaminants we originally sought refuge from, but with the growth of the health-food business, and corporate ownership of large health-food chains, exact duplicates of adulterated merchandise now line the shelves of the fancier, more efficient, more "packaged" shops. Look for the small, independently operated places filled with fresh produce, grains, herbs, and certified raw dairy *products,* or skeptically question your chain-owned health-food store proprietor regarding ingredients.

## Nutritional Autopsy: Adelle Davis

Adelle Davis did a great deal to alert people to possible deficiencies in their diet. She was a good pioneer journalist, but unfortunately her knowledge was incomplete, as is that of all people. Her books, however, read like and have been read like the Bible, often misleading people into absurd dietary pathways.

My purpose here is briefly to alert your skepticism to all dietary messiahs who propose to rescue you from "the sound of your own pulse in your ears" (i.e., your thoughts about life and death) with various magical diets and supplements. I will do this by speculating on the reason Adelle Davis may have developed the rare form of cancer that took her valuable life.

The poor woman died of plasma cell myeloma, a bone-marrow disease treated with metabolites such as folic acid *antagonists.* Having advocated and used rather high doses of folic acid, Mrs. Davis may have inadvertently induced the disease process herself. *Anti-*folates are believed to destroy cancer cells due to the fact that the malignant cells have much greater metabolic needs than normal cells (since they are growing so much faster than normal cells); thus, cancer cells mistake the anti-folates for folates, take them up, and thus deprived of folates they die. Perhaps the self-supplementation with high doses of folic acid tipped the delicate scale from a state of equilibrium? The point of this "autopsy" is to introduce caution in a field of self-medication which may *induce* serious disease

*Oversupplementation a Possible Hazard*

states if not properly planned. We are, none of us, immortal, nor is our advice infallible.

Having learned that vitamin/mineral supplementation has been with us since antiquity, and that various ethnic recipes advantageously condense nutrients, we examined the known micronutrients and speculated on their dosage. Various interactions which may affect nutrient needs were also explored and the hazards of oversupplementation underlined with a speculative "autopsy." Before looking at the therapeutic values of wine and beer, we must pay homage to the universal nutrient, water.

# 6 WATER: THE UNIVERSAL NUTRIENT

## What Lurks Within the Murky Well?

Today we live in an age in which pure drinking water is one of our most gravely endangered nutrients. Although the human body can exist for long periods of time without food, it is impossible to survive more than a few hours without water. Our bodies are composed of 60 percent water by weight and 75 percent by volume. The vital organs and all structural components in the body rely on a delicate fluid balance, which in turn is dependent on the purity of the exogenous water supply.

Of all the natural substances known to man, water is nearest to the universal solvent. Methods of filtration of our public drinking supply, however, are not adequate to ensure safe levels of particulate matter. Epidemics such as the European black plague, cholera, typhoid, salmonella, and infectious hepatitis were water-borne diseases. These scourges were a result of bacteria and viruses contaminating public water supplies. The oldest form of pollution known to man, human sewage, played host to these infections, which inevitably carried over to man's food supply.

*Modern Filtration Systems Inadequate*

In the late 1900s disinfecting agents, such as chlorine and hypochlorite in America and ozone in Europe, were added to public water supplies to kill bacteria and prevent the incidence of water-borne diseases. Even modern filtration systems, however, are not able to eliminate viral contaminants from public water.

*Water May*
*Carry*
*Carcinogens*

In addition to the refuse that is dumped in our water supply, we must contend with herbicides, detergents, radioactive wastes from atomic energy plants, and other carcinogens which may not be filtered out to a safe drinking level before dripping out of our faucet. Although the federal government has spent billions of dollars on water-quality research over the past two decades, the mandated legislation is not enforced effectively in many areas of the country. Because of the latency factor, a community may not experience an outbreak of cancer until fifteen years after it has been exposed to a carcinogen in the public water. Government officials sometimes dismiss the evidence as an epidemiological fluke, to avoid panic in the community. In 1978 national media coverage of an outbreak of leukemia in school-aged children brought officials from the National Center for Disease Control to Rutherford, New Jersey. All sixteen children who died of leukemia lived within a one-and-one-half-mile radius of Rutherford's elementary school. After several months of intensive laboratory investigation, no source was discovered. But Rutherford is located on the edge of the Hackensack Meadowlands, a great swamp where nearby industries dump toxic refuse. This is why the land flanking the New Jersey Turnpike is known as "Cancer Alley"; the Garden State has one of the highest cancer rates in the United States. The same industries that feed families with the breadwinners' wages also shorten the life span through exposure to carcinogenic substances. PCBs and THMs (chemical contaminants) are buzzwords in New Jersey, because people there have suffered inordinately from cancer of the liver and the lung.

A vast network of secrecy surrounds the formulas of the complex industrial chemical compounds that are polluting our water supplies. This makes long-term studies by regulatory agencies difficult, if not impossible. There are so many new compounds on the market that the Environmental Protection Agency cannot possibly keep up with the backlog of tests to determine their safety. It is more cost effective for industries to pay small fines for pollution violations than it is for them to invest millions of dollars in pollution-control equipment.

*Minerals in*
*Water*
*Insignificant*

Relatively little is known about the effects of long-term exposure to the numerous synthetic organic compounds in our water supply. Although trace minerals are necessary to ensure optimal nutrition, the quantities of beneficial trace minerals in our drinking water are sufficiently negligible to warrant the elimination of all minerals from the water supply. The essential trace minerals are far more abundant in fresh fruits and vegetables. Although the human body is extremely adaptable to all forms of environmental stress, when immunologic function is depressed, there is a greater risk of developing chemical sensitivities, such as allergies and cancer. These problems may certainly be aggravated by toxic soluble particles that pass through the filters of water treatment plants.

Pro-fluoridation spokesmen claim that the addition of fluoride to the public water supply at a level below significant toxicity will prevent the incidence of dental caries. The fluorine atom has nine electrons and voraciously acquires an extra electron in its ionic state. It binds to many beneficial minerals such as magnesium, potassium, calcium, copper, and zinc; by combining with these minerals, it forms mineral complexes that inhibit enzyme activity. According to a report on fluorides by the National Academy of Sciences, "fluoride inhibits many enzymes by formation of metal-fluoride complexes and by direct interaction with the enzyme and its substrate. Fluoride should be thought of as a general inhibitor of oxidative metabolism." Fluoride is not known to play any essential physiologic role; but specific illnesses, such as colitis, muscle spasms, neurological disorders, rashes, urinary problems, and gastrointestinal disorders have been traced to fluoride toxicity. Many older people suffer from the effects of fluoridation, especially when enzyme competency approaches marginal limits during aging.

*Fluorides Deadly*

Chlorine, used as a disinfecting agent, also has its dangers. Many studies have revealed a high correlation between chlorinated water and various cardiovascular diseases. Possibly worse than chlorine is the prevalence of asbestos in drinking water. In the mid-1970s asbestos exposure became a highly publicized issue when widespread cases of asbestos poisoning were reported among industrial workers throughout the country. Ironically, many water pipes consist of a combination of cement and asbestos; asbestos fibers are abraded and wash away in the water running through the pipes.

Many people have become aware of the risks of drinking unpurified water from their kitchen taps and have turned to bottled water. The projected sales for 1980 by the bottled-water industry are over $250 million—a big business indeed. This type of solution is not only expensive and inconvenient, but does not always guarantee an uncontaminated source of water. For example, even bottled spring water may contain asbestos, which may occur naturally in serpentine rocks where some spring water is drawn. In fact, federal labeling requirements do not spell out uniform regulations for a pure source of spring

*Bottled Water Unwise*

water. The bottled water that you buy in the store can be more dangerous than the sample in your kitchen faucet. The plastic gallon jugs are the heaviest item in the grocery bag and the containers are nonrecyclable.

# Types of Home Water Filters

Filtration has recently become a household word among concerned individuals. Among the various home water-purification systems we surveyed were sink-top filters, reverse-osmosis systems, deionizers, and portable home steam-distillation systems.

Sink-top home water filters are the best selling and least expensive item; however, one is hardly getting one's money's worth with these devices. The trouble with these low-cost filters is that disease-causing bacteria feed on the material that traps them and multiply within the water filter. Silver-lined sink-top filters may inhibit bacterial buildup, but also erode into the drinking water.

Reverse-osmosis systems separate tap water through a semipermeable membrane, so that there is a relatively higher concentration of impurities on one side. These units work by a delicate pressure system coming from the tap; but fluctuations in tap pressures may result in differences in quality of water output. Acidic water may cause the membranes of reverse-osmosis units to become ineffective. Similarly, alkaline water precipitates calcium compounds and clogs membrane pores.

Deionizers are only one step more advanced than water softeners. They remove positively charged ions such as calcium and sodium and negatively charged ions such as chloride or sulfate. Although they produce relatively pure water, the exchange medium is expensive and bulky and requires periodic maintenance. Although deionizers effectively remove inorganic, dissolved solids, they are useless against organic chemicals, viruses, and bacteria.

*Steam Distiller Best*

The most practical, cost-effective, and biologically safe system of home water treatment is the portable steam distiller. When water is boiled, all bacteria are killed. The water vapor that is captured is condensed and consists of pure distilled water. Since unwanted particles, such as heavy metals, are too heavy to rise with the steam, they are left behind in the boiling tank. Volatile gases such as ether and benzene are shunted out of a vent. And so, the home distiller is the best low-cost solution to all water contamination problems and is relatively maintenance free. As we try to cope with our increasingly polluted water supply, water distillers will become a necessary household appliance for modern twenty-first-century living.

# Radioactivity in Water*

Public waters may contain natural radioactivity, as shown below. These figures are relatively low, but often vary widely in the same region. For example, concentrations of radium-226 ranged from 3 to 36 picocuries per liter (pCi/liter) in well waters compared in Illinois, while radium-228 concentrations ranged from 0.9 to 7.9 pCi/liter.

*Natural Radioactive Elements Found in Water*

## Radium-226 and Radon-222 in Public Water Supplies (1962)

| Location | $226_{Ra}$ (PCI/LITER) | $222_{Rn}$ (PCI/LITER) |
|---|---|---|
| Austria (Bad Gastein) | 0.6 | — |
| Germany | 0.03–0.3 | $\leqslant 220$ |
| Sweden | 0.2–1 | — |
| United Kingdom: | | |
| Ground and surface water | $\leqslant 0.7$ | $\leqslant 200$ |
| Cornish waters | $\leqslant 2.4$ | $\leqslant 3,000$ |
| Devon waters | — | $\leqslant 13,000$ |
| United States: | | |
| Tap water | $\leqslant 0.2$ | — |
| Deep sandstone wall | $\leqslant 37$ | — |
| Surface water | $< 0.2$ | — |
| USSR: | | |
| Fresh water | 1 | — |

1 curie (Ci) = 1,000 millicuries (mCi)           1 microcurie ($\mu$Ci) = $10^6$ picocuries (pCi)
1 millicurie (mCi) = 1,000 microcuries ($\mu$Ci)

When reviewing the forthcoming entry on mineral waters, bear in mind that even these "healthful" drinks may contain radioactive elements: "Certain natural springs in areas of high soil levels of uranium and thorium have high levels of radioactivity originating from these elements" (Comar and Rust, 1973).

* Based on Comar & Rust in NAS (1973).

## Uranium-238, Radium-226, and Radon-222 in Natural Waters and Springs

| Location | $^{238}$U (pCi/liter) | $^{226}$Ra (pCi/liter) | $^{222}$Rn (pCi/liter) |
|---|---|---|---|
| **Austria:** | | | |
| Springs | $\leqslant 4$ | — | $\leqslant 10^5$ |
| **France:** | | | |
| Springs | — | $\leqslant 139$ | $\leqslant 10^5$ |
| **Germany:** | | | |
| River water | — | 0.07–0.8 | — |
| Springs | — | 0.07–18 | $\leqslant 10^3$ |
| **Japan:** | | | |
| Springs | $\leqslant 0.3$ | — | $\leqslant 7 \times 10^5$ |
| **Lebanon:** | | | |
| Springs | — | — | $\leqslant 6 \times 10^3$ |
| **United Kingdom:** | | | |
| River water | — | 0.01 | 0.2–0.3 |
| Springs | — | $\leqslant 12$ | $\leqslant 7 \times 10^2$ |
| **United States:** | | | |
| River water | 0.005–0.01 | 0.03 | — |
| Lake water | 1.7 | — | — |
| Groundwater | $\leqslant 40$ | $\leqslant 22$ | — |
| Springs | — | — | $\leqslant 3 \times 10^5$ |
| **USSR:** | | | |
| Springs and brooks | $\leqslant 3$ | — | — |

Note especially how high the concentration of radium-226 is in the spring waters of France ($\leq$139 pCi/liter). However, we are told not to worry about high concentrations of radon-222 in spring waters: "since this radionucleotide has only a mean life in the body of about one hour, the radiation dose is small."

*French Spring Water Questioned*

My question, in an age of bottled spring water (particularly from France), is what happens in our bodies during that one hour of exposure to the radioactive elements contained in the water? This is a question that remains disturbingly uninvestigated.

Of course, low levels of natural radioactivity may even prove beneficial. There is an interesting story of a Congolese tribe that treats cases of skin cancer by lying in the "magic mud" of a local river. Investigators found this mud to be uranium rich, but most fascinating is the fact that the locals "used mud only from those areas of the riverbank that were shown to yield the highest amounts of uranium" (Farnsworth, 1968). Here is another example of ethnic medicine in particularly sharp focus, and further reinforcement for my hypothesis that by observing various concepts of ethnic food and health, we may increase our adaptive strengths.

*Skin Cancer Treated by Folk Cure*

# Mineral Waters

Mineral waters are once again undergoing a revival of popularity. This is due in some measure to the widespread knowledge that our drinking waters are contaminated with various pollutants. On the positive side, people are drinking mineral waters partly as a substitute for alcoholic beverages in bar and social situations. It is a bridge for those who do not like to drink alcohol.

From ancient times mineral waters have been greatly valued as medicinal agents. The earliest Greek and Roman physicians advocated their efficacy in the treatment of many diseases, as can be found in the writings of Hippocrates, Aristotle, and Herodotus. Temples were even erected in proximity to mineral springs and dedicated to the healing Aesculapius. The early Egyptians, Jews, Arabs, and Mohammedans all used mineral waters in healing the sick, and Homer speaks of bathing and using the natural waters in healing. Pliny in his *Natural History* mentions a large number of mineral and thermal springs in different parts of Europe, and also speaks highly of their curative properties. For five centuries mineral waters were almost

*Mineral Waters of Historical Interest*

the only medicines employed in Rome, and the hot waters there have been in active use for drinking and bathing purposes for over two thousand years.

*Tiberias Springs Tried*

On a recent trip to Israel I tried the healing waters of Tiberias, where Jesus reputedly effected his dramatic water cures. I can only say that my intense anxiety was dramatically lessened by the treatment. This anecdote is not offered as scientific evidence but as testament to the validity of psychophysical interactions in therapy—a significant interaction in a book about food and health.

*Natural Sulfates in Mineral Water*

What should we make of mineral waters around the world? If in fact patients who went to take the waters for their cures were benefited by them, was it the water itself, or was it the rest that went along with the water? Was it the six or eight weeks that people took off from their otherwise hectic lives and the careful attention paid to them by physicians and other attendants—the good diet, good company, and great entertainments of the evening? I am not able to comment on that, but we should note that most or many mineral waters of the world, especially the more famous ones, contain high degrees of sulfates. It may be useful to compare the drinking water of a standard municipal system with regard to sulfate content, which is probably near zero, with the sulfate content of mineral springs which are known for their sulfur content.

As an example in the extreme, an analysis of the water at Marienbad springs, which were known as purgative springs, shows that these waters contain approximately 18 grams of sulfur per gallon of water. As a comparison, Vichy water in France contains approximately one-tenth that amount of sulfates per gallon, while the Sharon Springs in Schoharie County, New York, which are known as sulfurated waters, contain almost as much sulfate as the Marienbad water.

*Laxative Effects Cited*

From a scientific point of view, we would suggest that any beneficial effects experienced from these springs would most likely be due to the sulfates, which induce laxative effects. It is also possible that many of these waters contain trace minerals in significant amounts, especially in relationship to the American and European diets, which may be deficient in these minerals.

"Please do not introduce common sense into matters which have no room for it," says a character in the novel *Temptress* by André Maurois. Having attempted to do just this in a field of experts, often of differing opinions, I now direct your interest to a subject of little controversy between my clients and myself—alcohol and nutrition.

Spirits are what men will not do without.

—CHINESE PROVERB

# 7 ROOTS OF HEAVEN: ALCOHOL AND NUTRITION

Every healer I know, be they M.D.'s, Ph.D.'s, or lay-trained alternative therapists, all seem to drink or smoke. It is curious, though, the rationales one hears. One lady acupuncturist with an enormous clientele who smokes like a chimney insists that "it's what you *do* with the smoke" that determines whether one gets cancer or heart disease or skate through the tunnel of fumes. Another friend with an enormous reputation as an alternative physician drinks more heavily than anyone I've ever personally met, but before each glassful of "organic wine," which complements his vegetarianism, he takes handfuls of pills, mainly B vitamins, "to protect the liver." Rationalizations or reality? It matters not. So many of us are committed, if not addicted, to our vices, that we may as well live with them, taking our nutritional insurance as a hedge against disease. I am all for compromise, so long as our rationales are sound. Why not enjoy a bit too much good wine, if we know that a good dose of vitamin $B_3$ will protect our liver from fatty degeneration? Why not a belief system that allows us to smoke, even where the risk factors for our major causes of death gallop proportionately? Hell, we're all going to die, so we may as well live it up while we can, right?

Wrong. The quality of our life suffers after every indulgence. *Wine and Beer Advised* Not only do we satisfy the busy coffin measurers with every cigarette, but perhaps also reduce our optimistic vision as well. But when it comes to beer and wine, I am a firm believer that when free of additives and aged properly they have a definite place in sound nutrition. There is simply no justification for the overly Calvinistic and extremely simplistic attitude of abstention being proffered by too many self-declared nutritionists. If alcohol did not exist I would invent it, and judging by the way this simple compound has been greeted by the world's major religions, so would the rabbis and priests.

Since the beginning, man has sought relief from the tedium and vicissitudes of existence, and few recreational euphoriants, when taken in moderation, can match the safety factor of pure wine and beer.

# Wine

*Wine of Ancient Origin*

The discovery of fermentation may have been one of mankind's greatest breakthroughs, equal to fire and the wheel. Alcohol may have served as man's catalyst in evolution. In our leap along the evolutionary ladder, alcohol may have been our first major escape from the dangers and terror of early life on this planet. During moments of relative calm and relaxation, our distant ancestors certainly evolved as social animals.

Wine growing is one of man's earliest activities, predating recorded history. Ancient cuneiform tablets of the Sumerian culture refer to wine and the grape, as do later Babylonian cylinder seals and Egyptian hieroglyphics. The Bible speaks of wine and the grape in both metaphorical and literal senses, and today in the Jewish and Christian religions these symbols of health and renewal are still used as meaningful decorations for modern ecclesiastical objects. By praying to the Egyptian agricultural deity, Osiris, or by pouring a libation to the Graeco-Roman wine deity, Bacchus, or by thanking God for the fruit of the vine before a meal, man has endeavored to communicate with a being he believed guarded the earth's fecundity.

But wine is more than just a good-time drink famous for its tranquilizing properties. It has also been used as medicine, with specific wines from different regions being utilized for various complaints. While the specificity of different wines has been carried to a remarkable extreme in France, the American Wine Advisory Board recently published an interesting pamphlet, "Uses of Wine in Medical Practice," which outlined in general form its medicinal virtues. The following comments are derived from this publication.

## Major Indications

*Wine Is Medicinal*

Wine is to be recommended in the diabetic diet because alcohol is metabolized without calling upon insulin, and so dry wines serve both as a useful source of energy and as a valuable psychological factor in therapy. As a mild tranquilizing agent to counter emotional tension and anxiety, especially among the aged, wine is without equal. Disorders such as anorexia nervosa have been found to be ameliorated by the appetite-stimulating properties of dry wines. In cardiovascular diseases the tranquilizing and dilating properties of wine are well established. Since peripheral blood vessels are opened, this provides a mild prophylaxis against anginal attacks.

## Major Contraindications

The first type of patient who must *not* be encouraged to drink alcohol of any kind are those individuals who are incapable of using it without becoming dependent on it. More specifically, wine is contraindicated in the presence of ulceration of the mouth, throat, esophagus, stomach, or any kind of inflammation or irritation of these organs. It is also contraindicated with all other alcoholic beverages in gastritis, gastric hyperchlorhydria, gastric cancer, or upper digestive tract bleeding. All alcoholic beverages, including wine, are contraindicated in pancreatitis, and should be used with great caution in the presence of liver disease, acute kidney infection, prostatitis, symptomatic benign prostatic hypertrophy, genitourinary disease, or epilepsy. Finally, wine and alcohol in any form may react synergistically with such drugs as barbiturates, tranquilizers, narcotics, and other like agents. Pregnant women must abstain, owing to dangers to the fetus such as malformation, growth retardation, and impaired mental functioning.

*Wine Prohibited in Certain Complaints*

## The Chemistry of Wine

If you think that wine is a simple compound, made simply by squeezing grapes and allowing the juice to ferment in barrels and then filtering, realize that more than three hundred components have been isolated, not including the chemicals that are added to most commercial wines. These substances are produced as a result of the interaction between the microorganisms and the juice of the grape in the fermentation process. The great variations in composition of different wines are almost infinite, and depend on the type of grape used, the climate, the soil, the processes of fermentation employed, and the degree of aging. In general dry table wine is generally thought to be

*Wine Is Chemically Complex*

made up of 85 percent water, 12 percent ethyl alcohol, a bit of tartaric acid, and a few other compounds all contributing to its color, aroma, and taste.

*Wine Types Described*

Before describing the chemical ingredients, we should briefly describe different wine types. Red table wines are made from red grapes fermented in the presence of pigment-rich grape skins. White table wines are produced from white grapes, or from red grapes after the skins have been removed; and rose or pink table wines are usually made from pink grapes, or from red grapes that are fermented briefly in the presence of grape skins, and then with the skins removed. Champagnes and other sparkling wines are also table wines, containing approximately 1.5 percent carbon dioxide. Cocktail or dessert wines are ordinary wines to which brandy or grape neutral spirits are added to increase the alcohol concentration. These include sherry, port, muscatel, and related products such as vermouth.

*Little Sugar in Dry Wine*

All wines contain alcohols such as ethyl alcohol and others; carbonyl compounds such as acetaldehyde; acids such as tannic, tartaric, malic, citric, and phosphoric; esters such as ethyl acetate; and carbohydrates such as sugars. Dry red wines contain from 0.1 to 2 percent sugar. Dry white wines contain 0.1 to 3 percent sugar, while sweet wines are up to 4 to 5 percent sugar, and 15 percent or more in kosher wines. Cocktail or dessert wines contain about 2 percent sugar in dry sherry, 3 percent in medium sherry, 11 percent in sweet sherry, 12 percent in muscatel and port, 5 percent in dry or French type vermouth, and 15 percent in sweet or Italian type vermouth. The sugars present usually consist of glucose and fructose in about a 1 : 1 ratio. In addition, wines contain nitrogenous substances, amino acids such as glutamic acid, arginine, leucine, lysine, methionine, and at least seven other amino acids have been isolated.

*Red and White Wines Iron Rich*

Wines also contain vitamins in very small quantities, inorganic compounds such as potassium, sodium, magnesium, calcium, and iron, as well as trace minerals such as silicon, rubidium, zinc, manganese, aluminum, boron, copper, and others. Although iron is present in relatively small amounts, 80 percent of it is found in the ferrous form, and is rapidly absorbed. For this reason wine, especially port wine, is usually thought to have anti-anemic properties, but in actuality red and white table wines contain more iron than port does. But to keep it in perspective, two glasses of red table wine would provide only 20 percent of the RDA, 10 mg of iron, for an average male, and this is certainly not enough iron for treating iron deficiency anemia.

Alcohol interferes with the absorption and utilization of many nutrients, particularly zinc and magnesium. For this reason the consumption of nuts (unsalted) while drinking wine or beer is wise nutrition. Walnuts, for example, are a good source of magnesium, which tends to lend credence to this food combination once popular in English taverns.

*Eat Nuts While Drinking*

Also of interest is the fact that wine is generally rich in potassium, which may be significant to patients using diuretics. A recent analysis of California table wines showed that the potassium content averaged 1,260 mg per liter in red wines and 899 mg per liter in white wines. People on sodium-restricted diets should be aware that the sodium content of wine is generally low, but wines treated with ion exchange resins contain high amounts of sodium, a possible problem in states such as hypertension.

*Some Treated . Wines High in Sodium*

As a final note on the chemistry of wine, we should remember that wine more closely resembles gastric juice in pH than any other natural beverage. The average pH of wine is about 3.5, ranging from 2.8 to 4.1; the range for cocktail or dessert wines is 3.1 to 4.5, with an average of about 3.7. And so, in small quantities, wine increases salivation, stimulates the activity in the stomach, aids in the natural evacuation of the colon, while in larger amounts wine can seriously depress these functions.

*Wine Approximates Gastric Juice*

## Medical Claims for Wine

It has long been recognized that wine has a strong antibacterial property. This action is due to phenolic compounds, tannins, and anthocyanins. Wine has shown inhibitory action against various bacteria, including *Shigella dysenteriae, Salmonella enteriditis,* and *Staphylococcus aureus.* Plain grape juice, though, has a stronger antiviral effect than wine, again owing to the phenols that are located mainly in the skin and seeds of grapes. The development of arteriosclerosis may be inhibited by the regular use of wine, according to a recent study. In an interesting paper by Leary in 1931, it was stated that the regular use of wine can reduce the incidence of arteriosclerosis by as much as 50 percent. Experimental work has shown that wine can provide protection against excessive amounts of exogenous cholesterol; see Morgan, 1957. In Parkinsonism, a white table wine extract of Bulgarian belladonna root has shown highly satisfactory results in treatment. These results could not be duplicated when the extract was prepared with alcohol by itself.

*Wine Shows Antibacterial and Antiviral Activity*

*Wine*
*Metabolized*
*Without Insulin*

DIABETES  As mentioned earlier, dry wines serve as an excellent regular energy source in the normal diet of the diabetic, because wine is metabolized readily without calling upon insulin. Long before insulin had been isolated, the treatment of diabetes mellitus had been accompanied by the empirical use of wine: "Sixteen hundred years before the discovery of insulin, Aretaeus the Cappadocian described diabetes and used wine in its treatment" (Lucia, 1954). Wine can be utilized by diabetic patients being treated with insulin or oral hypoglycemic agents, and can be substituted for a calorically equivalent amount of fat in the diabetic diet without producing significant ketosis. Finally, it should be noted that more and more hospitals in the United States are beginning to serve wine to patients, a practice long known in Europe. Studies have repeatedly shown that the use of wine in hospitals lowered the overall number of complaints from patients by reducing emotional tension, fear, and anxiety, and at the same time stimulating appetite. As Galen put it, wine is "the nurse of old age."

## Heart Disease and Ethnic Drinking Patterns

There is little solid research to support the contention that rates of coronary heart disease are lowest in countries where wine consumption is great. Further, on examining the little evidence that exists, we can also conclude that the reason people have fewer coronaries in these Mediterranean countries is because they are less competitive than, say, Americans, the English, or Germans. That is, factors *other than* wine *or* fat consumption (beyond the diet) also play a role in the development of this and other diseases. Certainly attitude has a great deal to do with coronary heart disease, but this has been adequately treated by other writers and further comment is unnecessary.

## Chemical Additives in Wine

These hearty recommendations for the judicious use of wine are made in spite of the fact that many wines now contain a great number of chemical additives, many of which produce allergic responses in some people. Clients repeatedly complain to me of headache, fatigue, or nausea following the ingestion of certain brands of wine, but not of others. When brands are switched, such complaints often diminish. This led me to investigate the question of additives. It has not proven an easy search because industrial lobbies have recently successfully fought back a requirement that would have provided us with a list of ingredients on the label, including all chemical additives used before, during, and after processing. A check with the Food and Drug Administration produced no results; apparently people at the San Francisco office were completely unaware of any chemical additives in wine. Eventually, by tracking down a friendly person in the Bureau of Alcohol, Tobacco, and Firearms, I was able to get a list of chemicals that are permitted in the manufacture of wine.

Physicians and patients should be on the lookout for reactions to wine that may be the result of the additives and not the alcohol or congeners in the wine itself. By switching brands or, better still, trying an expensive imported wine, which often has fewer additives, you can determine if you are reacting to a chemical in the wine. There are additive-free wines available on the market, but they are very, very rare and very difficult to find. In a future publication I intend to investigate more thoroughly the question of untoward reactions from additives in wine, and in that book I will also list those wines available that are produced naturally and without any chemicals.

*Some People Allergic to Additives in Wine*

# Beer

Beer may have preceded bread, according to discussions at a symposium of the American Anthropological Society entitled "Man Once Lived by Beer Alone." The nature of fermentation and the intoxication arising from it were probably revealed to our ancestors purely by accident. Someone may have left a batch of half-chewed barley in a closed dish, still moist, then ate the altered leftovers a few days later and found himself delightfully changed. The accident was repeated; other villagers tried the stuff, and the art of brewing was gradually developed. From this early beer, this drink is now the most frequently consumed beverage in the world next to water. The healthful properties of beer in antiquity have since been diminished by highly commercialized, computerized brewing techniques; what was once a vitamin-rich beverage has long since disappeared in the average beer.

*Pure Beer Nutritious*

The recent scare about nitrosamines in beer served to warn us that an otherwise friendly beverage can often be replete with danger. It is interesting to note that the nitrosamines were not the result of any additives, but were generated during the

firing of the barley malt. Coor's beer, which had a zero level
of nitrosamines and was thus one of the safest beers tested,
enjoyed this zero level simply as a stroke of luck. It seems
that during the malting process the fire used to heat the grain
did not convert the naturally occurring nitrites into nitrosamines, as does occur in the malting of many other beers.

But there are other questions besides nitrosamines.

## Allergies and Beer*

*Allergens in
Some Beers*

A highly complex product like beer may contain small traces
of certain ingredients which may occasionally cause allergic
reactions. (Allergic reactions have even been seen with human
milk.)

A recent publication** lists many components not usually
associated with a glass of beer. People subject to allergic reactions might scan the following list for an offensive fraction:
carbon dioxide, fluoride, hydrogen sulfide, phosphate, sulfur
dioxide, calcium, copper, iron, magnesium, potassium, sodium,
methyl alcohol, ethyl alcohol, higher alcohols, diacetyl, acetaldehyde, lactic acid, hexoses, tannins, isohumulones, proteins,
ammonia, thiamine, riboflavin, pantothenic acid, pyridoxine,
nicotinic acid, and biotin.

## Additives in Beer

By far the most threatening fractions in beer are those con-
tributed by additives and preservatives. These have been given
wide coverage by the press recently. Representative Benjamin
Rosenthal (New York) has read a list of food and chemical
additives used in beer-making into the *Congressional Record*.

Seventy members of the House of Representatives have co-
sponsored a bill that would require brewers and manufacturers
of other alcoholic beverages to list all ingredients on their labels.
It is surprising that alcoholic beverages are at present exempt
from the labeling laws that apply to most other foods and
beverages.

Congressman Rosenthal, basing his comments on a recent
publication of the Center for Science in the Public Interest,
*The Chemical Additives in Booze* (Jacobsen, 1972), said "most

---

* The following material first appeared in Michael A. Weiner, *The Taster's
Guide to Beer*, (New York: Macmillan, 1977).

** C. D. Leake and M. Silverman, *Alcoholic Beverages in Clinical Medicine*
(Chicago: Year Book Medical Publishers, 1966).

of the chemicals are probably safe. However, some of the additives have not been adequately tested, and many individuals are allergic to certain others."

Much of the present concern with additives in beer grew out of a series of fatal heart attacks among heavy beer drinkers between 1964 and 1966. Mere alcohol was not to blame. It was discovered that cobalt sulfate, used at that time by several brewers to make thick, lasting heads, upset the metabolism of heart cells. Researchers believe that cobalt locks up alpha lipoic acid, which is needed by the vitamin thiamine to complete an essential reaction in a metabolic pathway of the Krebs cycle. The heart cells of the beer drinkers were thus destroyed by energy starvation.

*Heart Attacks Caused by Cobalt Sulfate*

While cobalt has since been banned in beer, consumer advocates insist that all additives must be listed on labels, to enable patients with known allergies to avoid those that affect them. To elucidate: even a little peanut butter may be fatal to individuals who are hypersensitive to peanuts. In the booklet *The Chemical Additives in Booze* it was reported that one such individual died after eating ice cream that contained peanut butter. Had the manufacturer been required to list the ingredient, the boy might have been spared his "accidental" death.

A list of some of the chemical additives that may be used in beer-making follows. While all brewers do not use all of these ingredients (or any of them for that matter—some brewers use *no* additives), many brewers continue to do so. Brewers in Germany, Switzerland, and Luxembourg are the only brewers in the world who are prohibited by law from using anything but barley malt, hops, water, and yeast in their beers. However, export beers of these countries are only required to meet the standards of the country that imports them. This means that, for example, a fine German beer, which is additive free in Germany, could enter other countries containing some chemicals. The only exception is Bavarian beers. Brewed to the strictest code in the world, beers from this region (a state of West Germany whose largest cities are Munich, Nürnburg, and Augsburg) are the same whether produced for the local market or for abroad.

*Beer from Bavaria, Switzerland, and Luxembourg Pure*

The addition of chemical agents to beer is an ancient practice. Adulteration has probably occurred from the time man began depending upon others for his foods and beverages. Public food inspectors were early assigned to check on manufacturers, and in 1309 English wine inspectors were required to take an oath to protect the public from unscrupulous wine makers.

## Chemicals Sometimes Used in Beer-Making*

| Name of Chemical | Purpose |
|---|---|
| Gum arabic, propylene glycol alginate (PGA), peptones | To stabilize foamy heads |
| Ethylenediaminetetraacetic acid (EDTA) | To prevent gushing when container is opened |
| Various proteases (papain, bromelain, etc.) | Chill-proofing (to dissolve particles that may cloud beer under refrigeration) |
| Ascorbic acid (vitamin C), isoascorbates, sodium bisulfite, sodium hydrosulfite, sodium metabisulfite, potassium metabisulfite | Antioxidants (prevent oxidation and subsequent loss of flavor and color) |
| Various enzymes | To speed up conversion of starch to sugar during malting |
| Heptyl paraben, hydroxybenzoate, diethyl pyrocarbonate | Preservatives |
| Caramel, FD&C Blue No. 1, Red No. 40, and Yellow No. 5 | Artificial colors |
| Acetic acid, adipic acid, anethole, benzaldehyde, citric acid, decanal, ethanal, ethyl acetate, ethyl isobutyrate, ethyl maltol, gentian extract, grapefruit oil, isoamylacetate, isoamyl butyrate, isobutyl acetate, juniper berries, lemon oil, licorice root, lime oil, malic acid, methyl anthranilate, nootkatone, octanol, orange oil, quassia extract, sodium citrate, sucrose, octaacetate, tartaric acid, terpineol | Flavoring and coloring |

* For further information see Thomas E. Furia, *Handbook of Food Additives,* 2nd ed. (Cleveland: Chemical Rubber Co., 1972).

*Government Lax*

The consumer must not assume that "the government is keeping an eye on them." The cobalt incident, the high probability that the common meat and fish preservatives, the nitrates and nitrites, are carcinogenic (they are used in pressed meats, frankfurters, etc., even while they are highly suspect), would indicate a lax governmental agency, more interested in protecting manufacturers from the demands of consumers than protecting consumers from unconscientious manufacturers.

The beer drinker must be made aware of the possibilities of contamination in his favorite brew (as well as in all foods and beverages). Accidents do occur. In London at the turn of the century six thousand people were affected by and seventy died from arsenic poisoning that was transmitted by contaminated beer. The contamination had originated not with the brewers but with the producers of brewing sugars—glucose and invert sugar. Nor was the brewing sugar producer himself at fault. He was using sulfuric acid that had been accidentally manufactured from highly arsenical iron pyrites.

# 8
# FLIES IN THE SLAUGHTERHOUSE

## Overcoming the Contamination of Our Food Supply*

*The Body Has Its Own Memory*

Man attempts to feed himself as though he were a cybernetic angel, when he is physiologically closer to the wolf than to the bird. Seemingly endless quantities of meat, sugar, white flour, salt, and chemical additives continue to take their toll while we pretend not to know. The food technologists, nutritionists, and physicians seem to conspire against self-knowledge—exploiting instead our absurd desire to transcend the zoological order. A vast array of synthetic foods attests to man's capacity for self-deception, a capacity in fact unknown elsewhere in the living world.

Feeding animals human treats is, of course, strictly prohibited at the zoo. Here we can see the origin of purely recreational eating. Candied popcorn must be mighty appealing to an orangutan fed in accordance with jungle laws. Yet the price for this nutritional transgression is paid by the deceived creature within a few hours; after eating sugared treats on Sunday many animals suffer from Monday-morning sickness, perhaps due to a mild hypoglycemia. We, however, have made a habit of deceiving ourselves and have so reinforced our distorted dietary ideas as to have conveniently forgotten the causes of our illnesses, when in fact too many are the result of our fabricated foods, sheer gluttony, and sedentary existences.

*Fad Diets No Solution*

We ourselves are not to blame. We are reinforced in our recreational dining habits by vast industries: food manufacturers, physicians (some of whom know better), teachers, and

* An earlier book of mine treats *all* categories of food additives, including naturally occurring toxicants. Readers interested in the broader picture may refer to *Bugs in the Peanut Butter: Dangers in Everyday Food* (1976).

authors of diet books who encourage us to make up for a lifetime of reckless living in only a few weeks of yet more reckless fad eating.

My answer to a lifetime of distorted nutritional attitudes is less extreme, yet more demanding. A *gradual* weaning from the overly processed, highly chemicalized foods and a shift to the more basic is demanded. Based upon years of clinical practice, I believe that this can be done once a true physiological portrait is established in the individual's mind: that we are living, breathing, feeling organisms with specific dietary requirements within parameters broad enough to allow for personal as well as cultural dietary preferences. Once we visualize where the stuff we put in our mouths goes and what happens to it, including those components that are indigestible, we will begin to seriously consider every morsel (before it is swallowed). *Gradual Weaning Suggested*

In not so ancient times flies in the slaughterhouse were a serious problem. Today rats won't *eat* refined flour, knowing perhaps more than we. Our problem is no longer food contaminated by rodents and insects, but rather the processing and preservatives. *Processing and Preservatives Now the Adulteration*

I am not the first to say that man's deviation "from the state in which he was originally placed by nature seems to have proved to him a prolific source of diseases." Edward Jenner's first paper on smallpox, in 1798, begins with this theme. How is it then that only a handful of us remember the truths that carry life from one generation to the next? Civilization depends upon a few truths, constructed through time, carried through new epochs. We must train ourselves to hear the words of our teachers, retreating through time and resting in universal truths, when confronted by modern questions. *Call for Return to Natural Diet*

"If you can hear what these patriarchs say, surely you can reply to them in the same pitch of voice" (Ralph Waldo Emerson). Has the human organism changed *biologically* since the dawn of recorded time? How then can the tinkerers insist that we live with a food supply that must render us ill? Have our digestive systems and cellular requirements evolved past the point of needing wholesome food? Why then are we told that ersatz substances, "fabricated foods," are wholesome? Wouldn't a sane population refuse these compounds as unworthy of consumption? Would a responsible government permit these items their place in commerce? *Man Not Adapted for Chemicalized Foods*

Apparently the scientists and their owners care little for themselves and the great throbbing mass of protoplasm that walks the streets. Most technologists encourage consumption *A National Malnutrition* of flavors and colors without food value in an attempt to deceive the people, to lull them into believing they are well fed, when in reality most of the people in the affluent nations are suffering from diseases of malnutrition!

*Diet Blamed for Much Disease*

"Americans are still the best-fed people in the world" is a saying commonly thrown in the face of those who raise the obvious question. But are we? Why are the rates of disease and suicide rising? (Over 50 percent of the people are being treated for a chronic disease. One out of three hospital beds is occupied by a "mental" patient.) Could it be that we are all starving to death from a devitalized diet in combination with deadly chemicals? Perhaps we know this instinctually but are too "well fed" to rise up in revolt?

*Scientists Termed Amoral*

Where are our scientists of conscience? We see a slippage from the high plane of vision established by former generations of scientific workers. Without much laboratory space, on bare essentials (fire, water, air, and the earth's elements), earlier workers achieved scientific advances of monumental significance compared with the trite, albeit "elegant," work of today. The DNA manipulators may be onto something, but confusing strands of life, mixing the cells of one animal species with another, may give our Dr. Sylvanas a sense of power while leaving the throbbing mass of humanity in the mire.

*Physicians Often Negligent*

And our physicians? How is it that in discussing euthanasia our "healers" no longer cite the Oath of Hippocrates? The answer is there: "I will give no deadly medicine to any one if asked, nor suggest any such counsel." Is abortion a new issue? Hippocrates dealt with this as well: ". . . and in like manner I will not give to a woman a pessary to produce abortion." Those therapists who defend their sins through clever arguments are refuted by words of the same Greek physician: "I will abstain from every voluntary act of mischief and corruption; and further, from the seduction of females and males."

*Hippocratic Oath Abandoned*

How is it that the Hippocratic Oath, a testament which withstood the trials of twenty-four centuries, is no longer part of medical training in too many medical schools? Do the ruling physicians fear the consequences of a moral generation of physicians?

If the human organism is so much as one hair different from its ancient stock, then the new food chemicals, derived not from nature, should produce worlds of unknown harmony.

Nature is profoundly impartial.
It cannot be persuaded by pampering,

nor dissuaded by scoffing.
It cannot be tempted by bribes,
nor influenced by injury.
It cannot be cajoled by flattery,
nor chagrined by slander.
Thus it is the most reliable thing in the world.

—LAO TZU

My skepticism has no bounds when it comes to various cult diets. Food additives, though, have no place in our inner ecology and here is where my skepticism ends. Many of the materials on the shelves of our markets may be potentially harmful. I am certain that many among my colleagues would state that the American food supply is the cleanest, purest, and most wholesome in the world. Are we certain? We are a long way from being certain.

Since World War II a chemical revolution has occurred in our food supply; thousands of materials are being added to the foods we eat. Originally materials were added to foods for the purpose of preservation. It was eventually recognized that some of these were toxic, and they were removed. More recently, not only has our food supply been altered to make it more attractive to our senses—changing its color, flavor, sound, and texture—but also substances are added to make the manufacturing process simpler, and to preserve the storage or shelf life of foods. At the same time, materials are removed from foods in order to accomplish the same end, including nutrients which are relatively unstable, but which are usually necessary for the body, such as polyunsaturated fats, and frequently with them, as in the milling of wheat, many vitamins and trace minerals are also removed. So we end up with a food supply that contains a tremendous number of added chemicals and a reduced number of nutrients; that is, the nutrient density, or the quantity of nutrients per unit of food which we eat, has been decreasing over time.

*Food Supply Altered*

Have not all of these chemical additives been tested for safety? The answer is, unfortunately not. During the early part of the chemical revolution, an addendum was made to the Food and Cosmetic Act of 1953 which required that any material that was added to food must be demonstrated to be safe before it could be added. At the time the law was passed, there were hundreds, perhaps at least a thousand, chemicals that were already being added to our food supply. Who was going to test the safety of each of these materials, and how was the safety to be tested?

*Many Additives Never Tested*

## Toxicology and Food

*Food
Toxicology Not
Adequate*

The science of toxicology utilizes techniques having to do with changes in organs which can be recognized in animals once they have been sacrificed and autopsied. Such classical toxicological techniques do not appear to be the proper approach to evaluating toxic materials—particularly things that may be injurious to health—in humans. It is well known that many substances that occur in food inadvertently, like the heavy metals such as lead and mercury, may cause serious damage, especially to the nervous system, at relatively low doses without killing the individual. This is particularly true in the growing child.

*Tissue Damage
Unnoticed*

Very frequently at levels where such lesions are produced when the substances are fed to animals, there is no visible sign of damage within the tissues. In other words, functional impairment may occur without any associated changes in the anatomy which are recognizable by any means at our disposal at present. As an example, it is now well known that one of the reactions to very low levels of lead intoxication in children is a decrease in the size of the visual fields—the development of tunnel vision and the loss of peripheral vision. The same type of defect can be produced in monkeys. After the defect is produced in monkeys, when the monkeys are sacrificed and their brains examined, there can be found no evidence whatsoever of any damage to the brain, yet we know that there has been damage because there has been a decrease of vision. We must be extremely alert to the fact that the testing of these chemicals which are added to our foods must be done in various species of animals and utilizing a variety of techniques, and must be done in most instances over several generations, to also pick up the possibility that these materials may be particularly injurious to the developing fetus, which is particularly susceptible to chemical or physical injury. Is such testing being carried out? Again, the answer is no, although it is required by law. There is apparently insufficient manpower, supposedly insufficient money, and possibly insufficient knowledge to perform an exhaustive study of every food additive, although the latter is certainly no excuse for the lack of testing, at least within the limits of our present knowledge.

*Governmental
Responsiveness
to Lobbyists*

The Food and Drug Administration, upon passage of this amendment to the Food and Cosmetic Act, had several choices. One was immediately to order the withdrawal of all food additives and to allow the various chemicals to be added only after suitable toxicological testing. Another option was to assume that the materials probably were safe, since there appeared to be no overt and reported manifestations of disease due to many or most of the chemicals in our food, and therefore to establish a grandfather clause, which would allow the addition of these materials to our foods, and then to begin a gradual process of testing. In the first approach the assumption would be that food additives are unsafe until proven safe. This would seemingly have been the correct and scientific approach. However, there arose a hue and cry from the food industry that this would be totally destructive of our food system, which was probably the main factor leading to the FDA's decision to take the second course.

How was the FDA going to decide which of the materials being added to foods were safe? The answer was the creation of the so-called GRAS list, which stands for substances "Generally Regarded as Safe." The FDA prepared an extensive list of the chemicals which they knew were being added to foods. Then they sent this list to members of the Institute of Food Technology, requesting that they state whether they thought these materials were safe or unsafe. There were also requested to extend the list with any additional chemicals which they knew were being added to food, and to indicate their opinion regarding the safety of these materials. If most of the responses supported the safety of a particular material, it was added to the GRAS list, and testing would be delayed indefinitely. Therefore many of the decisions concerning the presence of these chemicals in our foods were based merely upon the guess of a so-called "expert" in food technology. Yet these individuals often had no knowledge whatsoever of the actual or potential toxic properties of the material in question. *GRAS List Faulted*

Furthermore, most of the members of the Institute of Food Technology are employed in the private food industry; therefore most of the individuals questioned might be expected to reflect the bias of the food industry. Their bias clearly was one of attempting not to shake the boat, not to alter anything within the food system, and in this endeavor they have succeeded remarkably. *Toxicologists Biased*

So these materials continue to be dumped into our food, and no one, except the manufacturers themselves, knows the quantities of these substances which are present, for there is no law requiring that they divulge this information. The only labeling requirement is to mention all the ingredients, not their proportions. Only a few of the chemicals on the GRAS list have been extensively studied by modern toxicological methods and, disturbingly, a fair number of these have been found to be toxic and have been removed. Among these, for instance, are most of the artificial food colors. Formerly there were hundreds of artificial food colors which could be added to foods, but which were removed from the shelf. Now we are down to a very small number, less than a dozen, and even these are suspect and under further study.

## Maraschino Meetings

We all eat these glazed and shiny cherries in our ice cream, fruit desserts, cakes and pastries, even in our alcoholic cocktails. They are held out as special treats by smiling adults for attentive children. But few of us would give them to our neighbor's child after learning that:

*Adrenal Tumors from Red Dye #4*

1. The synthetic color used to make our maraschinos was *banned* from all foods on December 7, 1964, because feeding experiments with dogs produced cancer of the adrenals and bladder. When this synthetic color, FD&C Red #4, was added as 2 percent of their diets, 60 percent of the test dogs died.
2. The World Health Organization gives this color IV E, their *lowest* rating. This indicates that it has been found to be harmful and should not be used in food, under *any* circumstances.

It is unlikely that *anyone* would continue to eat these chemical time bombs if they knew these facts. But the question remains: why is this outlawed food color still being used? The *Federal Register* of August 19, 1965, holds the legal answer without presenting the scientific evidence.

*Industry Overrides Health Concerns*

Owing to pressures put forth by two trade associations (the National Cherry Growers and Industries Foundation, Portland, Oregon, and the Maraschino Cherry and Glacé Fruit Association, Cincinnati, Ohio), the commissioner of Food and Drugs, George P. Larrick, *amended* the original bill which banned FD&C Red #4.

As a result, this coloring was permitted ". . . in food only for the coloring of maraschino cherries . . ." as well as "in externally applied drugs and cosmetics *without* quantitative restrictions." This amendment was based on "studies" that followed the original ban. Attempts to get further details of these "studies" have not yet been successful.

Aside from the fact that no reference to the actual studies is made in the *Federal Register* (August 19, 1965), we learn that "notice and public procedure are not necessary prerequisites to the promulgation of this order because section 203(d) (2) of Public Law 86–618 so provides." This is mere rhetoric.

It is a depressing realization that after fourteen years of

work consumer groups successfully banned Red Dye #4, only to see their labors destroyed.

Here we have a known carcinogen in a very common food. This is a clear violation of the Delaney Amendment, which prohibits the use of *any* additive that produces cancer in *any* organism. Further arguments that there is not enough of this substance in maraschino cherries to induce harmful effects in humans fall apart when we remember that some children eat half a jar or more at one time. Even if the coloring is not toxic at the allowable levels, ingestion of many cherries would be potentially toxic, especially when we consider that the "gestation" period for many human cancers is generally at least twenty years.

*Maraschino Cherries a Time Bomb*

## Rainbow Poisons

Consumer fears of harmful food colorings first appeared in 1906, following the passage of the first Pure Food and Drugs Act. People were becoming alarmed about the new coal-tar colors just coming into use. Before this time, all colors added to foods were of natural origin. The first synthetic dye, mauve, was originally intended for coloring fabrics and other industrial products. It only took the rational but blind minds of a few people who wanted to cut costs to add this color to foods. Today, about 90 percent of all colors used in foods are synthetic. Their use is usually justified on the basis of being cost effective. Just recently, when Red #2 was banned, certain manufacturers claimed that this act would drive food prices up.

*Other Food Colors Dangerous*

But where do these coal-tar colors come from?

The term *coal-tar* is derived from the fact that the black viscous fluid obtained as a by-product in the manufacture of illuminating gas from coal was formerly the only technically important source of raw materials for the dyestuffs industry. Today these raw materials are also obtained from petroleum and by synthetic methods in such a pure form that their original source would not be identifiable. Nevertheless, even "pure" synthetic colors are to be avoided—especially when there is such a wide variety of natural colorings to choose from. In fact, there is presently a tremendous rebirth of use of natural colorings.

*Many Food Colors Derived from Petroleum*

Certification of a color by the government is *not* a guarantee of safety. A high percentage of the synthetic colors approved for use and available in the early 1950s *have since been prohibited from further use in foods* (e.g., Orange #1 and #2; Yellows #1, 2, 3, 4; Violet #1; Reds #1, 21, and 4, except for use in maraschino cherries, as you remember). Currently ten synthetic colors are approved for use in foods. Who can be certain that some or even all of these dyes will not one day be banned as a result of more exacting studies?

The addition of food coloring to enhance consumer appeal is a practice that dates back to antiquity and is not strictly an invention of modern food technology. The Roman scholar, Pliny, described the use of artificial coloring of wine more than two thousand years ago. Since the fifteenth century, when European explorers returned from the Orient with spices and dyes, food colors have become standard ingredients in processed foods. Both natural and synthetic food colors are used in processed foods to increase the acceptability and attractiveness of products.

*Coloring Can Conceal Damage*

But food coloring is often used to conceal damaged or inferior products. This form of deception is analogous to the used-car dealer who paints and waxes the body of a vehicle that has internal damage and puts it up for sale. The naive customer who purchases this unsafe and virtually worthless car has bitten into the flesh of a shiny red apple whose skin has absorbed a dose of red dye, but whose pulp may be bruised and laden with bacteria.

Approximately 100 million tons of carotenoid pigments are produced annually in nature. Carotenoids are natural dyes which are found in almost all fruits and vegetables, seafoods, dairy products, egg yolks, and in the plumage of birds. Carotenoids are not affected by the presence of reducing agents such as the antioxidant, vitamin C, and are not pH sensitive.

*Dyes Add Attractiveness*

Color is an important sensory phenomenon which stimulates consumers during their shopping. Unlike the sense of taste, which is not commonly perceived in the same manner, color is universally appreciated by all humans who have normal color vision. People are accustomed to colors as they appear in nature and will often reject foods that are inadequately colored. Consumers not only value the price and quality of foods, but also their attractiveness. Marketing experts try to offer what the consumer demands, regardless of nutritional value or safety. If certified dyes are removed, the colors must be retained that the consumer identifies with the products or they are left to rot on the shelves. Natural food colors that are currently available have technical difficulties in storage. They are often unstable, insoluble, or have low tinctorial strength, which may explain why synthetic dyes are predominant.

The phenomenon of sense perception, especially vision, governs behavioral responses, even though a visually appealing substance may be detrimental to one's health. Foods would appear dull and unappetizing without the accompanying attributes of flavor, texture, and, most important, color. All of these factors collectively form the basis of recognition. It is no accident that our favorite citrus fruit is named after its very color, orange. One cannot underestimate the psychological importance of color, especially the correlation between taste and color. The enjoyment of sweet foods is enhanced by stimulation of our visual senses as well as our olfactory senses. This is one reason why assortments of candies correlate to the painter's palette and help to satiate a pseudoaesthetic craving. We have forgotten the true colors of the rainbow, only preserving man's image of the heavenly spectrum in cold emblazoned reproductions. Even the wrappers magnify the bright colors of the contents, as a visual enticement to lure the tongue, nose, and eye into a collective cheap thrill which is rewarded by instant gratification.

But the refined sugar that corrodes the enamel of our teeth is not enough. White cane sugar is fine for dissolving in hot beverages, but is visually unappealing. We need the double-hit of a substance that is sweet to the eye as well as the tongue, and after the dye is cast, our ever-reliable liver attempts to detoxify the foreign color and allow it to pass through the walls of the bladder. In tests with laboratory animals repeated exposure to various food colors results in tumors of the liver and bladder. These stalwart organs can only withstand limited contact with carcinogenic substances before the cellular metabolism goes awry and then it is too late to restore proper immune function. *Bladder Cancer Related to Dyes*

The dangers of certain food colors were confirmed with tests using subcutaneous injections which induced sarcomas, a form of cancer growth. One of the first carcinogens used extensively in the laboratory was butter yellow. This substance produced hepatomas in the rat liver. In this case the carcinogenicity was limited to the liver, where the dye is metabolized. Residues of the well-known carcinogen 2-naphthylamine in Yellow OB and Yellow AB resulted in control of these substances. But we have only uncovered the tip of the iceberg. Red #2 is controversial not only as a carcinogen, but as a teratogen (fetal deforming). Other dyes are mutagenic and will not only influence the cellular metabolism of the persons ingesting the substance, but their offspring as well. *Butter Yellow Banned*

Presently in the United States the certified synthetic colorants include FD&C Red #40 (Allura Red AC), FD&C Red #3 (erythrosine), FD&C Yellow #5 (tartrazine), and FD&C *Which Dye Will Next Be Banned?*

Blue #1 (Fast Blue FCF). All of these synthetic colorants are permanently listed for food use. Those colorants which are provisionally listed and are still being tested include FD&C Blue #2 (indigotine) and FD&C Green #3 (Fast Green FCF). These colors are used widely in many nonessential foods such as desserts, soft drinks, candies, ice cream products, and snacks.

The key color among red colorants is Allura Red, which is basically orange-red but is not light sensitive. Tartrazine is canary yellow and Sunset Yellow FCF is orange tinted. Indigotine, which is a navy blue food dye, is rarely used for blue coloring because of poor light stability, but is used extensively for brown and black shades. Fast Green FCF is also not used widely because it is relatively expensive and gives an undesirable greenish-blue color.

The only four colors that are really desirable are Red #40, Yellow #5, Yellow #6, and Blue #1, which are for general usage, while others are used in more specific cases. Long-term toxicity studies are currently being conducted on carmosine, which is virtually identical to Red #2.

The three legally allowed nature-identical synthetic carotenoids are $\beta$-carotene, $\beta$ apo-8'-carotenal, and canthaxanthin. Colorants that are exempt from certification because they are natural and safe include the use of red beet powder, turmeric and turmeric oleoresin, grape skin extract (for beverage use only), annatto, cochineal extract and carmine, paprika and paprika oleoresin, saffron, and carrot oil.

## Nature's Rainbow

*Natural Colors Abound*

Other botanicals with color principles worthy of exploration include *blue:* campeachy wood (logwood); *brown:* catechu; *green:* chlorophyll; *red:* alkanet root, beet-red, Brazil wood, cochineal, black huckleberry, mallow flowers, pokeberry, sandalwood; *violet:* orchil; *yellow:* annatto, buckthorn berry, carotene, cudbear, curcuma root, Persian berry, p-turmeric, safflower, saffron, and yellowwood.

*Man Engineering His Own Demise*

As we stated in the introduction, toxins, as well as disease, have been with us since antiquity. We now know that man, in certain cases, is engineering his own demise in the name of frivolity. Nowhere is this more apparent than with the food colors, some of which are potent carcinogens, painted on a rainbow of foods. To overcome this internal pollution, be sure to read labels, avoiding any foods with artificial colors, selecting those undyed or colored from nature's rainbow.

To make a distinction between the unclean and the clean . . .
—LEVITICUS 11:47

# *9* KOSHER FOOD LAWS: TOWARD A REVISED INTERPRETATION

It is ironic that one of the world's earliest and most thoroughly developed food-purity systems is now so loosely interpreted as to permit the inclusion of health-damaging chemicals in products stamped "kosher" by attending rabbinical authorities.

*"Kosher" No Longer Assurance of Food Purity*

Surely dangerous additives have no place in foods considered "clean," even if they have been prepared according to laws of ritual purity. Kosher processed meats, such as salami and frankfurters, happen to contain unduly high concentrations of nitrites, a notoriously aggressive carcinogen. Modern dietary restrictions in Judaism should consider chemical additives as repugnant as the dreaded trichina worm, a too frequent passenger in pork products. Perhaps Orthodox Jews will reinterpret the above commandment to include food "preservatives" of questionable health value?

*Nitrites in Processed "Kosher" Meat*

I am aware, of course, of the argument that various food prohibitions have nothing to do with hygiene but are inspired by other considerations. There is the argument that animals are ritually slaughtered by specially trained rabbis—never the average person—to reduce the blood lust in man, and also to spare the animal pain, considerations quite separate from hygiene. This may be so; it is my intent, however, to include *more* hygiene considerations in the observance of *kashruth,* or the Dietary Laws—an "ethnic" system that has had a wide influence outside of the Jewish people. Modern "health-food" stores were inspired by the teachings of people like J. I. Rodale, an advocate of food purity who leaned heavily on his early learnings of the Hebrew Scriptures.

*Food System Also Related to Moral Principles*

My argument, of course, is not limited to eliminating nitrites from processed meat. The entire feeding chain of livestock must be reevaluated, and food pellets that contain growth hormones

*"Kosher" Beef Fed Hormones and Antibiotics*

135

and antibiotics which may end up in the finally "koshered" meat must also be reevaluated.

*Baked Products of Poor Quality*

Surely a box of cookies stamped with the highly coveted *U*—a seal granted approved foods by the ultra-Orthodox, and widely searched for by devout followers—these cookies should be made with ultra-wholesome ingredients, *not* refined bleached flour, sucrose, artificial colors, and artificial flavors, as are most such "approved" cookies presently made.

*Call to Incorporate Scientific Principles*

My suggestions should be seen in an amiable light. It is my intent to build on the tradition of Maimonides, who interpreted the laws, and, incorporating hygienic teachings he had learned, from the Greek healers particularly, created a set of health rules for his people and the world (see Chapter 3, "The Ethnic Factor").

It is not my intent to deny a people the food-purity system it praises as the greatest—especially since I belong to that people:

No consideration, however, will move me to set aside truth in favour of supposed national interests. Moreover, the elucidation of the mere facts of the problem may be expected to deepen our insight into the situation with which they are concerned. Sigmund Freud, *Moses and Monotheism*

*Kosher Food Laws Inherently Wise*

The Law of Moses, particularly as it applies to foods, has been well summarized by other writers and should be reviewed by those interested in the specific edicts (see, for example, Theodor H. Gaster, *Customs and Folkways of Jewish Life,* 1955, Chapter VI). As I wrote in an earlier chapter, there may be great wisdom in ethnic dietary laws, and we must reevaluate these teachings before summarily rejecting them as "old-fashioned" in an age of apparent sanitation.

*Prohibited Foods Often Contain Toxins*

To give one example, "clean" aquatic creatures, fit for food, are those possessing both fins and scales. Excluded, therefore, are lobsters, crabs, oysters, shrimp, and all other shellfish, as well as eels. What is the possible wisdom of this law, in a world of shrinking resources, particularly of the type of high-quality protein found in the prohibited seafood? We must look at the evidence of seafood toxicants discovered only recently.

## Shellfish Toxicants

Besides their ability to concentrate potentially toxic minerals, shellfish are also responsible for many cases of poisoning caused by toxic substances ingested from marine algae on which the shellfish feed. These shellfish poisons are usually resistant to heat, so cooking does not eliminate their toxicity; nor are they broken down by human digestive systems.

One particularly virulent form of paralytic poisoning from shellfish begins with almost immediate numbness of lips, tongue, and fingertips, spreading to legs, arms, and neck, and progressing to general muscular incoordination. Within two to twelve hours, depending on the dose, the victim dies from respiratory paralysis. If one survives twenty-four hours, the prognosis is usually good and there are no permanent effects.

Until fairly recently this form of shellfish poisoning remained a mystery. Shellfish in a given area might be edible for generations, then suddenly would become extremely poisonous and remain so for one to three weeks, after which they would again be safe for human consumption. In 1937 a group of scientists identified the organism responsible, a microscopic plankton in the waters around the mussel beds along the California coast. When mussels ingest this plankton, they become poisonous until the toxin has been destroyed or excreted, which takes one to three weeks. When environmental conditions are favorable, these poisonous plankton thrive and enter the mussels through the food chain. When the concentration of these plankton reach a certain level, the water takes on a reddish-brown color, known as a red tide. *Shellfish Often Unsafe*

The poison from these California mussels, known as saxitoxin, was isolated in 1954. It is an extremely potent neurotoxin, with no known antidote. The Klamath Indians used sugar pine gum as a folkloric remedy, but the gum has not been proven experimentally to be an effective antidote. *Saxitoxin Found in Mussels*

Related species of toxic algae producing the same kind of poison are found in the shellfish of many of the coastal waters of the North Atlantic and North Pacific.

Another shellfish toxin, called oyster or asari poison, is produced by another group of microscopic organisms that infest the oysters of Japan. This toxin causes fatty degeneration of the liver and kidneys, and has been responsible for hundreds of cases of poisoning and a large number of deaths in the Hamana Bay area of Japan. The toxic principle has been isolated and is quite stable to heat.

It is very difficult to detect these poisons in shellfish, since there is no difference in appearance between poisonous and nonpoisonous specimens. The usual method of detection is the microscopic monitoring of the water near shellfish beds; when *Shellfish Poisons Difficult to Detect* the toxic microorganisms reach detectable levels in the water, the shellfish are tested by administering them in extract form to mice and observing whether the mice die. Government agencies in this country carry out such testing periodically between May and October; if the shellfish become poisonous, warnings are posted and publicized.

*Kosher Food Laws of Universal Interest*

We could expand this reinterpretation of biblical dietary laws and elucidate other "reasons" to explain them, perhaps even to justify following them whether or not we are "believers." Of course many of these comprehensive dietary laws make no sense whatever from an objective sanitary perspective. For example, animals that "part the hoof" and "chew the cud" (cows) are not necessarily cleaner than those that are single-hoofed, such as camels. Food taboos, such as the above, incorporated into the Laws of Moses, may have served to cohere the Israelites and separate them from their neighbors as such taboos do in other ancient and contemporary primitive societies.

*Other Religions Share Similar Prohibitions*

The Code of Manu, an ancient Hindu tract, also proscribes animals that do not "part the hoof," and all birds of a carnivorous nature. This proscription is also found "in the compendia of ancient 'Aryan' laws attributed to the sages Apastamba and Vasishta" (Gaster, p. 203). Similar food taboos in contemporary primitive groups have been shown.

*Self-Discipline Inherent in Teachings*

The point is, these dietary rules all serve to impose a general self-discipline on their followers, a form of food authoritarianism enjoying a revival in our "scientific" world, where various components found *within* foods have largely replaced the gross anatomical differentials of the Bible.

Where the pig, the crow, the squid, and like creatures are forbidden by the Hebrew dietary laws, saturated fats, sucrose, and chemical additives are the "unclean" or forbidden in the ideology of internal health of rational man.

*Reinterpret Kosher Food Laws*

We must respect various ethnic food preferences and prohibitions, and attempt to rationally interject scientific knowledge so that dangerous food additives and sucrose are gradually rejected as "unclean." I support tradition but urge my religious friends to eliminate dangerous components of their foods, developed and introduced long after biblical laws were written.

# Book Three
## MORNING
## BRIGHTNESS

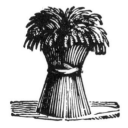

Eventually we have come to a conception of health and disease by which the two merge into each other, when men eat in order to prevent disease instead of taking medicine in order to cure it. This point is not stressed enough in the West, for the Westerners go to see a doctor only when they are sick, and do not see him when they are well. Before that time comes, the distinction between medicine which nourishes the body and medicine which cures disease will have to be abolished.          —LIN YUTANG

# 10 FOOD AS MEDICINE

## People Are Like Plants

Reverse anthropomorphism may be healthy for an all-too-egotistical creature such as man. When we look at trees and other plants, why do we seek *their* similarities to *man* when a reverse perspective may yield equally useful medical truths?

Visiting an organic farmer in Utah who raises cherries and peaches for allergy clinics worldwide, I was moved by the extreme health and vitality of the orchard. I learned that my friend had purchased the eight-thousand-plus trees only a few years back and he had already managed to improve them. "How did you do it?" I asked on the long drive out of Provo Valley to the Salt Lake airport. "Weren't any fertilizers or pesticides needed?" This vigorous, religious businessman/farmer told me a secret which I at once recognized as a key to health.

"You begin by improving the soil, using natural fertilizers, and slowly the trees themselves gain a new resistance to insects and internal degradation." The huge chain of neck-bending mountains, the site of America's Zion, stood witness to my profound confirmation of an ancient principle: treat the person, not the illness.

*Treat the Person, Not the Illness*

By introducing synthetic drugs for too many complaints, the physician weakens the natural resistance to further onslaughts of ever-present disease-rendering organisms. By neglecting to include whole, natural foods in their diets, too many people weaken themselves to infection, weakness, fatigue, and eventually grand ailments. Vitamins, minerals, and other supplements may be likened to chemical fertilizers; they are useful for producing a bountiful harvest in the short run (i.e., vitality and "health"), but will not substitute for a total reconditioning

*Protoplasm Likened to Soil*

of the "soil," our protoplasm. Only a steady, persistent approach to noncontaminated foods, plant, *and* animal products for those who prefer them, together with other healthful modalities, such as regular moderate exercise, can maintain our health.

But all of us fall ill sometimes, even the strongest. When this occurs, it is wise to evaluate the diet and life changes before proceeding with any therapy. And then, as in ancient times, with an inner dialogue, perhaps some fasting, food is our best first aid.*

# No Dietary Absolutes

*Be Skeptical of the Pedestrian Practitioner*

There are no absolutes in nutritional science. The field is in flux and the state of the art today will be rapidly superseded by tomorrow's research findings. Nevertheless, some diet-health relationships are well documented, understood, and operational, if not yet accepted by the majority of the medical community. As in all fields of science we must look to the more dynamic scholars for our leads, retaining our skepticism without assuming in advance that our more daring colleagues know too little to be of practical value for our daily practice.

Aldous Huxley has written, "Life must be lived forwards but can only be understood backwards." Medical nutrition is an ancient art, only now being rediscovered and "reprogrammed" to the needs of contemporary disease patterns and styles of living. As science confirms many nutritional ideas of the past which were thought to be of little value to the modern physician, we begin to understand the wisdom of the ancients. In the past, diet was employed *first* for most medical problems, drugs being reserved for those conditions not responsive to dietary manipulation.

*Food Is Medicine*

Food *is* medicine, as the ancients taught. But we now also know that food and drink, being composed of complex chemical structures, are capable of acting like drugs when in our bodies. When we further consider the limitless number of possible interactions between nutrients, we see why our consideration of diet becomes a *primary* concern, something to be looked at during our initial visit to a physician.

Before proceeding to *specific* dietary regimens for various disease states, we must withdraw to the larger picture, lest we err in concluding that diet, by itself, is king.

* Of course, crisis situations demand immediate therapy, at the extremes of technological capabilities.

# Undoing the Medical Model

Looking at the question of diet for disease states in the long-term evolutionary, biological, and psychosocial perspective, we see that man has somehow managed to survive, multiply, and inhabit all niches of the ecology of the world, and to do so while eating the most varied diet types of any known animal species. In view of this historical perspective, and the highly successful evolution of man, can we now think that we have the knowledge to tell individuals how and what they should eat when ill? This does not mean that I am a total nutritional nihilist when it comes to the question of diet and food. There are certainly areas of wisdom that we have achieved within recent years, as well as over the centuries.

*Man's Evolutionary Success Not an Assurance of Health*

If we trace the historical dietary treatment of almost any disease, we find that there were once wide variances from so-called normal diets during illness. We now find that the tendency of mainstream dietary therapy is to utilize diets that are not far different from those diets that people eat in order to maintain health! This has largely happened because of standardization of hospital procedures, especially menus, strictly out of cost considerations.

*Cost Rules Diet Therapy*

This has happened, unfortunately, because nutrition has fallen into the *medical model* and been taken over by it. The general medical philosophy is that diet or food is something to be prescribed; i.e., you prescribe for illness, you prescribe for health, you prescribe for the maintenance of health. Physicians are continually advising people what to do. In the case of nutrition, the medical model tends at times to become quite disastrous, owing to the fact that most physicians have very little knowledge of nutrition and seem to have an aversion either to referring people to professionals who have this knowledge, or communicating with such nutritionists themselves.

*Meals Prescribed Like Drugs*

One of the most regrettable scenes in the average clinical setting is of the doctor taking a preprinted diet from a drawer and handing it to the patient, somehow expecting that this will in some way influence the patient in any but an adverse manner.

*Preprinted Diets Useless*

Around the turn of the century (a time when many of us would like to believe things were still reasonably sound), patients generally ate wholesome, farm-raised foods, and the staff of life was still whole-grain bread. In those days diet lists were already being given to people for illnesses like diarrhea, constipation, diabetes, gout, obesity, and rheumatism. Nutritional science has moved forward, sideways, and backward since the beginning of the century. But the gastrointestinal tract of man, while an extremely adaptable, versatile mechanism, has not changed by one mitochondria since then. We still require wholesome food, on a regular basis.

The ingestion of food, however, is not merely a biological phenomenon, which I have repeatedly emphasized, but it is likewise a psychological phenomenon, and it is probably as important to the individual to feel that the food he is receiving is something with which he has an acquaintance and will not bring harm.

*Most Hospital Diets Unrelated to Health Principles*

This desire for familiar foods explains why so few people question hospital diets, and why so few refuse to eat menus prepared by dietitians. The food looks "balanced" from a purely archaic "four food group" perspective and is therefore perceived as safe to eat. Unfortunately most hospital diets are utterly unsound, usually catered by the same chain-food businesses responsible for America's malnutrition.

# The Hospital Diet

*Malnourishment Caused by Hospital Diets*

The majority of patients who are hospitalized, even if they have not come to the hospital malnourished, develop malnourishment within seven to ten days of hospitalization. This has been recognized as one of the most serious problems of hospitalization. Instead of people becoming revitalized, they become progressively run down and malnourished; in fact, the malnourishment can extend to the point where they become *more* susceptible to various diseases, especially the highly infectious. The immune system often becomes incompetent, and also hospitalized patients frequently suffer actual muscle atrophy. A considerable amount of the so-called posthospitalization weakness or asthenia is not only due to bed rest but is a manifestation of malnourishment that occurs within the hospital. This is totally inexcusable, but it is related to the poor knowledge of nutrition on the part of physicians and dietitians. That the nurturance of the individual and the building up of his or her own defenses are probably the most important factors in recovery, seems to be lost sight of.

Technological advances such as total parenteral nutrition have saved many lives. It is now possible to feed an individual who is unable to take food by mouth by placing a small plastic catheter in a large vein close to the heart. By this method sufficient purified nutrients can be given so that not only does the patient not become malnourished, but he can be restored to a normal state of nurture, even being made obese on occasion!

But the phenomenon of malnutrition in many hospitalized patients is a fact, first recognized by mothers of young children suffering from leukemia. These observant mothers were often told that chemotherapy had removed all evidence of cancer; yet children were dying in their mothers' arms! Obviously this made no sense, and it was the mothers who recognized that their children were dying of starvation. The therapeutic modalities of antineoplastic or chemotherapeutic agents and intensive radiation had led to a total lack of appetite and an inability to hold food by mouth. These children would not eat, or if they ate, would frequently vomit, and they gradually faded away. While the disease was responding to the miracles of modern medicine, the children were dying of that age-old scourge, starvation. It was the mothers who insisted that something be done to reverse this process, and here total parenteral nutrition was introduced to carry the child through this transition phase when the child was unable to eat.

*Mothers First Observed Malnutrition*

Children with leukemia now often survive, and we can begin to speak of cancer cures through the miracle of modern medicine. But this has only occurred with the realization that it is also necessary to supply the *total* nurturance of the child, including food and love.

And so, while the hospital diet is now recognized as grossly inadequate, few hospitals can be found where natural foods are served as a substrate for clinically effective menus. Nevertheless, we can treat ourselves with food, perhaps even inducing our physicians to do likewise.

*Natural Foods Are a Substrate of Recovery*

While the scope of this book does not permit an encyclopedic listing of all diseases responsive to nutritional therapy, I have selected a number of conditions where diet and disease may be strongly related. This information is not meant to be used for diagnosis or treatment, but is offered for consideration by physicians *and* patients, working together.

*Major Ills and Diet*

First I will treat some disease states at length (allergies, heart disease, mental disorders, and viral diseases), and then make brief comments for other disorders with nutritional modalities (cancer and dietary relationships are treated as a separate chapter).

## Allergies (to Food)

*Almost All Foods Disagree with Some People*

As we saw with fava beans and milk products (in "The Ethnic Factor"), many people may be affected negatively by specific foods. Up to 20 percent of American schoolchildren may suffer from some form of allergy (Arbeiter, 1967), while many adults have discovered that they "break out," "itch," "flush," and so on when they eat chocolate, strawberries, tomatoes, nuts, eggs, milk, fish, grains, crustaceans, and many other foods! Quite a range of problem areas, in an age of starvation.

*Limits to All Fields of Inquiry*

We will deal directly with *known* allergies in food, but I must first enter a note of caution, if not outright skepticism. So many people claim to be "sensitive" to so many foods that we must first define terms, and set limits on the discussion in order to preserve reason in a field rapidly developing unreasonable expectations of miraculous cures for long-standing nonspecific complaints.

*Allergy Related to Immune System*

WHAT IS AN ALLERGY?    Allergy, which signifies an altered reactivity to some external stimulus, or antigen, is a branch of the broad field of immunology, which is the study of the immune system, or that complex system occurring in many organs which protects the body against invasion by organisms and "protects" us against many nonliving substances, particularly if they are protein in nature.

The immune system is extremely complex, and operates at different levels. Some of the immune mechanisms operate only at the tissue level. Others are humoral; that is, the protective mechanisms circulate throughout our blood, seeking to do away with the foreign invaders. We generally have no perception of this constant protective activity which is going on in our bodies. But from time to time, for reasons that are still quite unclear, the body reacts rather violently to certain of these foreign materials, with resulting symptoms, the most common being symptoms of hay fever, asthma, and eczema. This state of altered reactivity which causes the patient discomfort is spoken of as an allergic response or allergy. The manner in which the antigens trigger these reactions may be quite clear at times, as in the case of pollens causing hay fever or certain specific inhalants leading to allergy, but in many instances it is difficult to find the offending agent. This is particularly true in cases of long-standing skin allergies such as eczema. Various procedures have been devised in the past to test extracts of suspected material that might cause these reactions, by applying them to the skin and then scratching through the skin, or injecting them intradermally, and seeing if a skin reaction appears. This form of testing is still useful in some types of allergies. Recently more sophisticated techniques have been devised, which rely upon the identification of the reactions of certain part of the immune mechanism, which can develop a high specificity to certain of these external contaminants or allergens. Some recent inroads in the testing of specific parts of the immune system have resulted in the discovery of a class of immunoglobulins, IgE, which are likely the "skin-sensitizing antibody in man" (Jaffé, 1973).

The allergic response is a complicated problem because it may be due not only to the presence of the allergen itself, but also be dependent in part on the condition of the host. Exposure to cold, fatigue, stress, possibly multiple antigenic exposures, all tend to predispose the individual with the allergic diathesis, or tendency to develop allergies, to be more likely to have an allergic attack in the presence of the offending allergen.

*Food Allergy Multifactorial*

In the case of food allergies, aside from the use of IgE immunoglobulins, to attempt to identify the offending agent the classical technique has been the so-called elimination diet. The individual is placed on the simplest type of diet that will maintain his or her state of nourishment for a period of seven to twenty-one days. If the symptoms subside, this is presumptive evidence that the patient is suffering from some type of food allergy. Gradually various foods are introduced and if the allergy returns when a given food is added, this is presumptive evidence of an allergy to that specific food or some component of it. In order to prove that this is so, the offending food is again removed, and if the individual again shows improvement and/or recovery, this is considered positive clinical evidence of an allergy to the food.

*Elimination Diet Described*

Now, both this technique and the question of the symptom complexes which may be caused by food allergy, as well as the frequency of occurrences of food allergy, are the subjects of great debate. Some people claim that except in children food allergy is an extremely rare disease; others believe that it is one of the most common diseases of modern man. The latter group, those in the "clinical ecology" camp, claim that food allergy can lead to a whole host of symptoms, and that virtually any organ or organ system can be affected. These range from the so-called tension-fatigue syndrome through headaches, nervousness, indigestion, abdominal pain, head-

*Symptoms Described*

aches, migraine, learning disability, behavioral disorders in children, and a whole host of other complaints.

*Placebo Effect Possible*

There is no doubt that placing people with many of these diseases on an elimination diet does lead to an amelioration of symptoms. As a nutritionist I believe that if the therapy is efficacious there is no reason why the patient should not remain on that therapeutic regimen as long as it can do him no harm. However, the question is, has the technique of the elimination diet, restoration of food, elimination again, and a corresponding appearance and exacerbation of symptoms proven that we are dealing with a "food allergy"? The answer from a scientific point of view must unfortunately be an unequivocal no. The above sequence does not constitute sufficient scientific evidence. Again we can refer to the placebo effect, the effect of being involved in the therapeutic regimen, and the knowledge that a considerable number of people will improve on any therapeutic regimen. To prove that we are dealing with a true food allergy would require a rather complex experimental design, and to our knowledge no one has yet attempted to perform such studies. Furthermore, as I have emphasized repeatedly, the tremendous cultural and psychological meanings of food, both to the individual and to the family, may so affect the dynamics within the individual or the family structure as to lead to all types of changes and relief of many symptoms, particularly those associated with stress.

*Caution Required*

I again wish to emphasize, however, that because a given therapeutic measure has not been "scientifically proven" does not mean that it cannot be useful and should not be employed for a given individual. I only mean to sound a note of caution that treatment of "food allergies" is not a panacea for many of the illnesses of which they are considered the cause, and that not every individual who has one of the many illnesses that have been attributed to food allergy should necessarily expect a response from an elimination diet.

More recently other techniques have also come into being for testing for food allergy. One which some workers claim is an effective test for allergy is to place extracts of various foods dropwise under the tongue. It is alleged that within minutes, or even seconds, after applying the material, the allergic individual will manifest the allergic symptoms, if challenged with the proper food. Many of these same physicians claim that at one dilution the material may be used for testing purposes, but that at other dilutions a single drop may neutralize all of the allergic manifestations and cause them to disappear, and the individual will no longer be allergic to the given material. This likewise has not been tested under rigorous scientific methods.

Amines, enzymes, and gluten are all well documented as food allergens, but may not be adequately understood.

AMINES, VASOACTIVE IN FOOD   Certain compounds found naturally in foods cause a dramatic increase in blood pressure when injected into mammals. Tyramine, dopamine, and norepinephrine are found in foods, and people suspecting sensitivity to any of the foods listed below should bring the fact to the attention of a nutritionist or allergist, or simply avoid the offending dietary component. *Blood Pressure Raised by Certain Foods*

Many people claim sensitivity to pickled herring, various cheeses, certain wines and vinegar, and meat extracts. These foods likely contain the vasoactive amine tyramine, as a result of the fermentative processing or due to microbial action during *Tyramines in Herring, Cheese, Wine, Vinegar, etc.*

## Vasoactive Amines in Plant Foods

| Plant Substance | Amine in μg/gm or μg/ml* | | | | |
|---|---|---|---|---|---|
| | SEROTONIN | TRYPTAMINE | TYRAMINE | DOPAMINE | NOREPINEPHRINE |
| Banana peel | 50–100 | 0 | 65 | 700 | 122 |
| Banana pulp | 28 | 0 | 7 | 8 | 2 |
| Plantain pulp | 45 | — | — | — | — |
| Tomato | 12 | 4 | 4 | 0 | 0 |
| Red plum | 10 | 0–2 | 6 | 0 | + |
| Red-blue plum | 8 | 2 | — | — | — |
| Blue plum | 0 | 5 | — | — | — |
| Avocado | 10 | 0 | 23 | 4–5 | 0 |
| Potato | 0 | 0 | 1 | 0 | 0.1–0.2 |
| Spinach | 0 | 0 | 1 | 0 | 0 |
| Grape | 0 | 0 | 0 | 0 | 0 |
| Orange | 0 | 0.1 | 10 | 0 | + |
| Eggplant | 0 | 0 | — | — | — |
| Pineapple juice | 25–35 | — | — | — | — |
| Pineapple, ripe | 20 | — | — | — | — |
| Passion fruit | 1–4 | — | — | — | — |
| Pawpaw | 1–2 | — | — | — | — |

FROM Lovenberg, 1973.

* A dash means the food was not tested for this amine, 0 means that the level of the amine was below the detection threshold, and + indicates the material contained a trace of the amine.

aging or storage. The foods listed below should be studied for possible dietary elimination by people showing a sensitivity, and must in all cases be avoided by patients taking MAO inhibitors, such as isocarboxazid, nialamide, phenelzine sulfate, and tranylcypromine, drugs used to treat depression. Serious hypertensive states have resulted in such patients, because of the interaction between the drug and tyramine in foods.

*Histamine Also Vasoactive*

Other vasoactive amines are present in certain foods and people who "react" to sauerkraut, chocolate, stored fish, wine, beer, or other fermented or stored foods should consider the presence of histamine as a possible culprit.

As Lovenberg has aptly summarized, the clinical significance of vasoactive amines in foods is that:

(a) Amine metabolites in urine may lead to erroneous interpretation of certain clinical tests; (b) an amine-rich food is a distinct health hazard to an individual receiving a monoamine oxidase inhibitor; and (c) the amine may itself be toxic.

*Antidepressant Drugs Interact Rudely with Certain Foods*

A dangerous rise in blood pressure has been noted in a patient taking a MAO inhibitor who also ate as little as 20 grams of cheese, while headaches are often the result of histamines in common foods, particularly fermented beverages (wine, beer, sake, etc.).

ENZYMES    Another overlooked area of food allergy is the enzymes found in certain foods which produce toxic effects. For example, the carp, sardine, and some shellfish may contain vitamin $B_1$–destroying enzymes, known as thaminases (Jaffé, 1973).

*Common Grains Contain Gluten*

GLUTEN    Some people are unable to eat grain products containing gluten. This disease state, which may be considered a food allergy, is variously called *celiac disease* or *nontropical sprue*. In celiac patients a normal food protein produces a toxic effect where the absorption of other nutrients is impaired, often leading to advanced malnutrition. A biopsy of the jejunum is required to properly diagnose the disease (the villi are missing or small, the mucosa is flat); but the treatment is simple. All grains containing gluten must be avoided. These include wheat, rye, oats, barley, and buckwheat. It is actually the gliadin fraction of gluten that injures the intestine of sensitive individuals; but when all dietary sources are eliminated, the intestine will heal, eventually returning to normal function.

A true gluten-free diet, simple in principle, is complicated by the fact that grains are often used as the starting material

## Foods Reported to Contain Tyramine of Probable Microbial Origin

| Food Substance | TYRAMINE ($\mu$G/GM) |
| --- | --- |
| CHEESE: | |
| Cheddar | 120–1,500 |
| Camembert | 20–2,000 |
| Emmenthaler | 225–1,000 |
| Brie | 0–200 |
| Stilton blue | 466–2,170 |
| Processed | 26–50 |
| Gruyere | 516 |
| Gouda | 20 |
| Brick, natural | 524 |
| Mozzarella | 410 |
| Blue | 30–250 |
| Roquefort | 27–520 |
| Boursault | 1,116 |
| Parmesan | 4–290 |
| Romano | 238 |
| Provolone | 38 |
| BEER AND ALE | 1.8–11.2 |
| WINES | 0–25 |
| MARMITE YEAST AND YEAST EXTRACT | 0–2,250 |
| FISH: | |
| Salted dried fish | 0–470 |
| Pickled herring | 3,000 |
| MEAT: | |
| Meat extracts | 95–304 |
| Beef liver (stored) | 274 |
| Chicken liver (stored) | 100 |
| MISCELLANEOUS: | |
| Soya | 1.76 |

FROM Lovenberg, 1973.

in many foods, such as white vinegar, whiskey, salad dressing, root beer, and hundreds of packaged products. Consult your nutritionist or physician for a complete diagnosis and proper diet if you suspect that your symptoms (nausea, vomiting, diarrhea, gas, etc.) are related to this category of foods.

## The Mystery of Heart Disease

*Vitamin B$_6$
May Save Your
Heart*

Owing to the great number of years I've invested in reducing my fat intake, particularly of cholesterol-rich foods which I've always loved (eggs, shrimp, meat, cheese), only to learn that merely reducing these food fractions is not enough, but that increased intakes of various nutrients, particularly vitamin B$_6$, may be required to offset the deranged fat metabolism that may underlie the disease process, I am only willing to offer the suggestions of Dr. Roger Williams. This famed biochemist, the man who named folic acid and first synthesized vitamin B$_6$, offers the best theoretical framework presently available for understanding how to prevent a heart attack. This is particularly true for those of us who run a higher risk of developing this condition because of genetic factors, but it is becoming increasingly important for the general population, including the "nutritional rogues," of whom fewer members are visibly apparent with each new decade.

Why our more distant ancestors did not die of heart attacks as frequently as we do now can be speculated upon from many different angles. The commonly heard arguments are that they led less stressful lives (where, in poverty-striken Europe or Asia?), were more active physically (often not the case among the scholarly class, who generally did not die from this cause at an early age), or they ate differently (which I heartily support). The question now is, how can we modify our diet to reduce our risk of sudden death from this disease, or to slow the process in our children? We will answer this pressing concern after first reviewing the workings of the heart, and the overall picture of the disease.

THE GREAT PUMP    From a physiological point of view we can explain the action of the heart as that of a pump; the only function that the heart performs is pumping the blood through the body. Obviously this is an extremely important function because if it ceases, even for a few minutes, the lack of nourishment—oxygen—to the brain, leads to death of the brain, a condition that is often considered to be the equivalent of legal death, even though the heart may resume beating subsequently. Heart failure leads to a series of events, including attempted adaptation mechanisms of both a hormonal and neurological nature, the end result of which is an increase in the amount of circulating blood which the heart must pump (which it is unable to do), and an increase in the amount of salt that the body retains.

The treatment for this condition is to decrease the salt burden on the body. This can be accomplished in one or both of two ways. The first is to decrease the amount of salt ingested. The other is the use of medication that in a sense poisons the kidney so that the kidney excretes excess amounts of salt. The difficulty with the latter method, however, is that in the process of "poisoning" the kidney, not only does the kidney lose the type of salt intended, namely sodium, but it also loses other types of nutrients and salts, particularly potassium. These nutrients must be replaced, either by the ingestion of foods containing large quantities of these materials, which are found primarily in bananas and other fruits and fruit juices as well as vegetables, and/or the provision of these salts in the form of solutions or pills. The need for repletion of other salts does not occur if the condition is treated by dietary means. But many people will not eat diets that are extremely low in salt, and frequently the failure is so severe as to necessitate a very marked decrease in salt intake. And physicians would frequently rather use a medication than modify a life-style pattern such as eating, so the tendency has been to rely on these medicinal agents, or diuretics, although the same effect can be obtained without complications through nutritional manipulation merely by reducing the amount of salt ingested.

*Heart Failure Requires Regulation of Salt*

The other aspect of heart disease which is now in the throes of a serious debate has to do with the greatest killer of all in our society: atherosclerosis. Death often results from the formation of a clot on this fatty deposition, or atherosclerotic plaque, which occurs in the arteries of the heart, and which leads to a blockage of the blood flow to the heart. This condition is commonly known as a heart attack, or myocardial infarction. Once the myocardial infarction has occurred, the tendency of virtually all treating physicians is to place the patient on a special diet.

*Heart Attack Followed by Strict Diet*

I often ask: if the patient is placed on the diet at this point in time, why was he not placed on the diet, or the diet at least suggested to the patient, long before the atheromatous plaque formed? It is well known that it takes many years for the atheromatous plaque to form. The question is, what is the relationship between the formation of the plaque and diet?

*Fat Not Simply Related to Heart Disease*

Over the course of the last number of years it has been quite vociferously asserted that there is a very high correlation between certain fats in the bloodstream and the incidence of development of myocardial infarction and/or atherosclerotic plaques. As we learn more regarding this relationship, we find that it is not as simple as we had previously thought. The correlation is found among a variety of these fats, some of these fats when elevated being associated with a higher incidence of heart disease, while other fats when elevated are associated with a lower incidence of arteriosclerotic heart disease. Certain of these fats, and especially cholesterol and triglycerides—which when elevated are associated with an increased incidence of arteriosclerotic heart disease—can be significantly modified in most individuals by dietary manipulation.

The general recommendations for this type of dietary change are as follows. To accomplish a reduction in either or both of these fats, the individual is advised to decrease the total amount of fat consumed; generally to decrease the amount of protein, particularly meat protein; to increase the amount of unrefined cereals, whether grain products or potatoes; to decrease the amount of refined sugars in the diet; and probably to increase the amount of vegetable oils or fats in the diet. In fact, this last objective is usually accomplished automatically if one decreases the amount of meat, which is primarily fat and not protein, and decreases the amount of fat in the diet; for in increasing the amount of cereal grains in their natural form, one automatically increases the amount of polyunsaturated fat or vegetable-fat oil, because natural grain products are a fairly good source of these oils, which are removed in the milling process. This diet additionally tends to increase the amount of fiber ingested. It appears that fiber itself will cause a lowering of these blood fats by some mechanism, and also fiber may act as a protective mechanism in detoxifying and protecting the bowel against noxious agents that may cause diseases such as bowel cancer. Finally, the presence of fiber, which tends to attract moisture, eases the work of the bowel in expelling the fecal material, and may diminish those complications of constipation that arise so frequently in Western man.

*Heart Attacks Declining*

In the case of cardiovascular disease, it is interesting to note that over the last several years there seems to have been a tendency for a *decrease* in the incidence of, and particularly deaths from, heart attacks. This cannot be attributed only to the introduction of the newer techniques of caring for patients with heart attacks in coronary care units, because the percentage of change in mortality is much greater than can be accounted for by the number of patients hospitalized in these units. One explanation seems to be that there has been some modification of diet in a fairly high proportion of the American population, and this change in diet includes a reversal of some of the factors that we have spoken of as having been associated with affluence. The main changes have been alterations in the amount of fat, and particularly an apparent increase in the amount of polyunsaturated fat in the American diet. Also, a reduction in the amount of sugar has occurred, particularly in the coronary-prone population. Only a much more precise epidemiological study than we now have available will be able to answer this question of dietary change in a conclusive manner.

THE MIRACLE OF PYRIDOXINE    Having stated previously (see "Overcoming the Famine Within") that dietary fats per se may not be as significant in the development of coronary heart disease as previously assumed, I will reiterate that the nutrient pyridoxine (vitamin $B_6$) is particularly important in preventing the development of atherosclerosis and CHD. This conclusion is primarily based on the literature review of Dr. Roger Williams, who cites studies worldwide which tend to corroborate his viewpoint.* To put it in his words, "A derangement of essential fatty acid metabolism and of cholesterol ester metabolism in particular may be a most important factor in the etiology of atherosclerosis." And further, "It may very well be that pyridoxine deficiency is the limiting factor in this metabolic abnormality."

The many references cited by Dr. Williams serve to convince me that he is right, and I am particularly impressed by the Russian study of "forty-eight atherosclerotic patients with hypercholesterolemia" (high blood cholesterol). Thirty-one of these patients were shown to have "very low plasma levels of the coenzyme forms of vitamin B-6," and Williams suspects that "the subjects may have had an excessively high pyridoxine requirement, or may have subsisted previously on a diet deficient in B-6, or, alternatively, may have been unable to absorb the vitamin at its normal concentration in the diet, and responded only to therapeutic doses (100 milligrams per day)."

*Some People May Require 100 mg of Vitamin $B_6$ Daily*

This is a perfectly plausible explanation and would also explain why people in industrialized nations who eat pyridox-

*$B_6$ Destroyed by Food Processing*

* See especially Dr. Williams's explanations of references 1–73, pp. 245–303, in his notes to Chapter 5, "Protecting the Hearts We Have," in *Nutrition Against Disease*.

ine-deficient diets also often suffer elevated cholesterol levels, atherosclerosis, and the type of heart attacks that are related. Packaged foods have much lower amounts of vitamin $B_6$ than do fresh foods, and a deficiency of this critical nutrient is part of the national malnutrition I mentioned earlier. More than 70 percent of this vitamin is lost when whole wheat is converted to white flour; sugar and fat are devoid of it; and cooking losses further deplete this critical vitamin from the typical Western diet. In 1969 the average per capita availability of pyridoxine per day was just a shade above 2 mg (!), and this figure does not reflect losses during cooking or waste. Even people who think they eat "well," taking cereals, fruits, vegetables, milk, and other foods with little vitamin $B_6$, evidence signs of deficiency (Bogert, Briggs, Calloway, 1973).

*Many Ethnic Dishes Rich in $B_6$*

Looking at a list of good food sources of this vitamin in a standard university text, I am impressed by the number of foods that are (or were) frequently part of many ethnic dishes, including whole-wheat flour, walnuts, sunflower seeds, soybeans, salmon, brown rice, raw green peppers, roasted peanuts, filberts, chickpeas, lima beans, bananas, avocados, chicken, and raw fish (a frequent part of traditional Japanese meals).

*Supplement Recommended*

In an age of deethnicized, highly processed, overcooked foods, the safest course is supplementation of this essential nutrient. Alcoholics, pregnant women, the aged, and people on certain medications (see "Overcoming the Famine Within"), as well as those with various genetic and pathologic conditions, have even greater needs for vitamin $B_6$. Those with heart attacks in their family history must consider their needs for this vitamin carefully, and eat the foods listed above in greater quantity. The suggested vitamin/mineral formula listed in Chapter 5 provides 3 mg of this vitamin daily, an amount adequate for most people, but more is required by others, as noted above.

In later chapters, particularly "At the Nutritionist," and "A Strategy for Daily Dining," specific methods of analysis for and ingestion of this vitamin and other nutrients are clearly described.

## Mental Disorders (Depression, Hyperactivity, Hypoglycemia, Schizophrenia)

Brain chemistry is perhaps more complicated and less charted than any other bodily activity. To presume we know how to correct all mental conditions on a definite basis is not my posture. What follows is highly speculative and largely anecdotal. But the therapeutic regimens are incorporated here because of the success cited by reputable investigators and the relative margin of safety associated with the recommended nutrients.

TRYPTOPHAN: A NATURAL SEDATIVE AND ANTIDEPRESSANT In the past few years the National Institute of Medicine reported a marked decrease in the number of prescriptions for hypnotics and barbiturates for the treatment of sleep disorders. The number of accidental deaths reported in patients who combined these medications with alcohol has made many physicians more reluctant to satisfy their patients' requests to refill their prescriptions for sleeping pills. A similar danger of drug potentiation exists with the tricyclic antidepressants among people who do not limit themselves to social drinking. Although both the minor tranquilizers and tricyclic antidepressants have useful functions in the treatment of insomnia and mood disorders, a substitute drug which is a natural building block of proteins, L-tryptophan, has brought about equally promising results without the associated dangers of drug potentiation.

One of the oldest remedies for insomnia comes in the form of homey advice: warm milk before bedtime, as needed. L-tryptophan is a naturally occurring amino acid which is present in high concentrations in milk and other foods. In studies conducted at the National Institute of Mental Health, patients receiving L-tryptophan for five consecutive nights experienced an increase in total sleep when compared with placebo controls. Another important consideration is that L-tryptophan does not interfere with the rapid-eye-movement stage of sleep, as do the barbiturates and most minor tranquilizers, and does not produce drowsiness upon awakening. Thus, foods richly supplied with this amino acid are a good way to treat insomnia, anxiety, and depression.

*Warm Milk a Remedy for Insomnia*

Recently there have been a number of publications concerning the use of L-tryptophan in the treatment of psychiatric disorders. This amino acid is readily absorbed through the blood-brain barrier, where it is converted into the neurotransmitter serotonin. Serotonin has a number of biological effects such as in treating insomnia, obsessive-compulsive disorders, endogenous depression, perceptual schizophrenias, and as an anorexigenic agent in bariatric medicine.

In recent years tryptophan has been used in relatively high doses (5 to 7 grams at bedtime) in the treatment of endogenous depression. There have been a number of studies suggesting that depression is a result of a biochemical defect in the synthesis of serotonin from tryptophan. Depressed patients who expe-

*Common Amino Acid Alleviates Depression, Sleeplessness*

rience the common symptom of early-morning awakening are aided by high doses of tryptophan. The most potent form of tryptophan is in combination with vitamins $B_3$ and $B_6$, which are necessary constituents of the enzymes that convert it to serotonin. Dr. Alec Coppen, director of the Neuro-Psychiatry Research Laboratory in Surrey, England, has used low doses of imipramine, the original tricyclic antidepressant, in combination with tryptophan and found a clinically significant improvement in the patients studied. Tryptophan does not carry the risks of side effects and can serve as a valuable adjunct to a minimal dose of tricyclic antidepressants. Its potential for dependence and tolerance is very low, or possibly nonexistent, in contrast with other unnatural sedatives. L-tryptophan is an unlikely candidate for accidental death or suicide because of its relatively nontoxic effects, and is available in tablet form on most vitamin shelves and can be purchased without a physician's prescription. The only side effect of tryptophan is a mild sensation of drowsiness, which is why this natural drug is primarily indicated at bedtime.

Although tryptophan may increase the appetite of a self-starving individual, weight gain is not experienced in patients who have a tendency toward becoming obese. Psychobiologic studies of obsessive-compulsive disorders, which are characterized by dwelling on thoughts that one cannot reject, repetitive questioning, and an inability to make decisions, found that high doses of L-tryptophan ameliorated these symptoms after one month of therapy.

Tryptophan is one of twenty-two amino acids, and is found in many proteins, as about 1 percent of the total. Foods particularly rich in this antidepressive amino acid are steak, fish, eggs, chicken, soybeans, cottage cheese, milk, mixed nuts, beans (baked), and soya protein. Many ethnic recipes contain some of these foods and are the wisest method of incorporating this natural treatment for the disorders outlined above.

*Bladder Cancer Warning*    I must caution readers against taking this or any other isolated amino acid in large doses. Animal studies suggest that certain tryptophan metabolites may act as cocarcinogens, and worse, elevated levels of these metabolites have been detected in about 50 percent of bladder cancer patients studied (Yoshida, 1971). If we are to reject saccharine and other potential carcinogenic foods, then we must be consistent, and avoid *all* supplements of possible toxicity, taking increased amounts, if needed, via whole foods and adaptive recipes that maximize their concentration.

HYPOGLYCEMIA: IS IT REAL?    A recent survey by the U.S. Public Health Service revealed that almost 50 percent of the people questioned claimed that they were suffering from some variant or symptoms that were ascribed to hypoglycemia. Yet many physicians believe this condition is nonexistent. What is hypoglycemia, and how do we identify its presence?

*Many People Now Believe They Suffer from Hypoglycemia*

Shortly after the discovery of insulin in 1924, Dr. Seale Harris noted that some people not taking insulin, when given a glucose tolerance test (a test in which a large load of glucose or corn sugar is given) experience some symptoms similar to insulin reactions during the subsequent six-hour period. Some of these individuals showed evidence of high blood sugars during the first three hours of the test, succeeded by low blood sugars during the next three hours. He first called this condition hyperinsulinism, that is, overproduction of insulin, later changing it to dysinsulinism, or an error in the production of insulin by the body. He attributed this phenomenon, currently referred to as reactive or functional hypoglycemia, to a delay in the release of insulin followed by excess insulin release and an inadequate response by the anti-insulin mechanisms that are unable to compensate quickly enough to prevent the excessive fall in blood sugar. In fact he related two factors—one a rapid fall in blood sugar, and the other a fall in blood sugar to levels *below* those expected following administration of glucose—to the production of symptoms.

The term *functional* or *reactive hypoglycemia* is appearing more and more frequently, not only among the lay public but among clinicians as well. The condition has been "documented," in that certain individuals display glucose tolerance curves marked by an initial period of hyperglycemia or high blood sugar, followed by a more rapid than typical fall, and succeeded by a level of blood sugar *lower* than those seen in so-called "normal" individuals after glucose loads.

The primary question is whether some of the many rather nonspecific signs and symptoms attributed to mild or even moderate hypoglycemia can be posited as the source of the numerous somatic complaints associated with this so-called disease. Among the symptoms that have been gathered from various sources are the following: dizziness, fainting, blackouts, headaches, fatigue, exhaustion, drowsiness, narcolepsy or falling asleep, muscle pains and cramps, cold hands and feet, numbness, insomnia, nightmares, irritability, crying spells, restlessness, inability to concentrate, excessive worrying and anxiety, depression, forgetfulness, illogical fears, suicidal tendency,

*Symptoms Can Be Frightening*

tremors, cold sweats, inner trembling, incoordination, convulsions, fast or noticeable heartbeat, blurred vision, gastrointestinal upsets, lack of appetite, hallucinations, delusions, loss of sexual drive, and more recently, severe mental illness of every kind, ranging from mild or moderate psychoneurosis to severe depressions and schizophrenia. It is perfectly clear that almost any of us have at one time or another suffered, or are currently suffering, from at least one of these symptom complexes, but does this mean that the symptom complexes are really due to hypoglycemia?

Diets that presumably counteract hypoglycemia are frequently prescribed and recommended by many popular writers. But the issue continues to provoke controversy, with many experts contending that true functional hypoglycemia is rare and that most such diagnoses are merely faddish explanations. Some investigators such as Cahill of Harvard have pointed out that 23 percent of the population exhibit blood-sugar levels that would be diagnosed as hypoglycemia, without symptoms, when a glucose tolerance test is administered. Another author, Yeager, entitled one of his papers, "Non-Hypoglycemia as an Epidemic Condition." Therefore a more adequate set of criteria for functional symptoms of hypoglycemia are necessary for the clinician to provide a tool for understanding its etiology. Although severe hypoglycemia, usually induced by insulin or insulin-manufacturing tumors, produces virtually unmistakable manifestations including tremulousness, convulsions, coma, and even death, many of the other symptoms that have been attributed to so-called reactive or functional hypoglycemia are open to considerable question.

*Is This a Disorder or Symptomatic of Other Problems?*

The scientific controversy as to whether reactive hypoglycemia is a true disease, or merely a support for diagnoses of many psychoneurotic symptoms, remains unresolved, and is fueled by reports from both orthomolecular psychiatric literature, which frequently lends support to "miraculous" cures with dietary therapy, and the popular media. On a nationally televised program a probation officer claimed that low blood sugar was at the root of many of the problems encountered by the parolees under her supervision. A judge was so convinced of the truth of these claims that an "antihypoglycemic diet" was incorporated into the legal apparatus governing these particular parolees. The judge presented a choice of diet or jail.

Even with increasingly stringent criteria being sought for the diagnosis of clinically significant hypoglycemia, the relationship between the level of blood sugar, or the rate of fall of blood sugar, and symptom complexes remains extremely ambiguous. The general approach to the problem is to institute a therapeutic regimen, and if the therapeutic regimen succeeds in ameliorating or removing the symptoms, the diagnosis is considered established. However, as we have frequently mentioned, a change in diet is not only associated with a change in nutrients, but is also associated with a marked change in the psychocultural milieu in which the patient operates, and this latter may be as important as the alteration in the nutrient content of the food. However, the therapy for the alleged hypoglycemic individual can certainly lead to no harm when judiciously implemented, and in many instances may lead to a marked improvement in nutritional status. Many individuals complaining of hypoglycemia have histories of having been on high sugar intakes for long periods of time, and many scientists, particularly clinicians who deal with these people, attribute the development of this so-called hypoglycemia condition to the excess strain placed on the pancreas, leading to a condition in which there is a delay in insulin release because of the high sugar content of the average Western diet.

The therapy advanced for this condition is a diet low in refined carbohydrates, relatively high in fats and proteins, and consumed approximately six times daily in order to even out the usual elevations of blood sugars that occur after any type of meal. We now know that the type of carbohydrate is also important in modifying the glucose tolerance test. The elimination of sugar, and substitution for sugar of complex natural carbohydrates such as unrefined cereals, vegetables, and root crops such as potatoes, results in a marked lowering of blood sugar in normal individuals as well as diabetics and an alteration in the shape of the curve of individuals suffering from hypoglycemia. In addition to this, the type of fat that is taken should be carefully considered. Emphasis should be placed upon the *avoidance* of high saturated fat. Attempting to correct this condition with a high-protein diet derived primarily from meat sources, which will give a high saturated fat content, is *not* to be recommended. Coffee, tea, cocoa, chocolate, and other caffeine-containing drinks, *and* alcohol, must be avoided to stabilize the blood-sugar curve and prevent rapid swings in mood. Dividing our feedings into approximately six meals per day, or three meals and three snacks, is totally adequate in most instances to control the hypoglycemia, and hopefully, for those who believe that there is a relationship between this hypoglycemic reaction and the symptoms, to control the symptoms as well.

*Six Smaller Meals a Day, Sugar, Caffeine, and Alcohol Restriction Recommended*

CHROMIUM AND THE GLUCOSE TOLERANCE FACTOR    Researchers have investigated a dietary factor derived from brewer's yeast, which is rich in chromium and aids in the proper use of glucose and carbohydrate metabolism. Many people think of chromium as the raw material from which shiny bumpers of automobiles are molded and not as an essential mineral that is a natural constituent of many vital enzymatic pathways, including nucleic-acid metabolism and insulin-responsive amino-acid transport. Although chromium is considered a micronutrient, which is needed in only minute amounts, the absence of this essential trace mineral may be a factor in maturity-onset diabetes. Pure inorganic elemental chromium is not readily absorbed and serves no nutritional function. However, the complex that is formed between trivalent chromium and the amino acids glycine, cysteine, and glutamic acid form a configuration that is known as glucose tolerance factor. Most of the chromium in processed foods is lost and needs to be replaced in supplementary forms.

*Diabetes Mellitus May Be Alleviated by This Trace Metal*

Chromium is necessary for normal fat metabolism as well as for maintaining insulin balance. In its bound form chromium activates insulin and helps to convert sugar into usable glycogen or fatty acids. When insulin levels are high, glucagon is depleted, even though it is essential in the metabolism and utilization of fats. An absence or deficiency of glucagon may clog the arteries with fat deposits and accelerate the development of atherosclerosis. Thus this trace mineral has a definite function in the prevention and treatment of diabetes. In the chapter "At the Nutritionist's" the hair analysis used for detecting low levels of chromium is discussed.

HYPERACTIVITY IN CHILDREN   Severe malnutrition in both men and animals retards both the production and synthesis of cells in the nervous system as well as the connecting processes known as axons and synapses. Rats fed a diet deficient in serotonin exhibit a heightened sensitivity to painful stimuli. As previously noted, these effects can be reversed by feeding a diet adequate in tryptophan. Similarly, rats deficient in another dietary substance, choline, exhibit subnormal levels both in the blood and the brain of another important transmitter of nerve impulses, a material known as acetylcholine. Further, it has been found that human beings on certain types of psychotherapeutic drugs for long periods of time develop a strange type of incoordination known as tardive dyskinesia. This condition can virtually be cured by the administration of choline, perhaps by restoring the normal balance of this material in a critical part of the brain.

Another important suspected relationship between dietary factors and behavior is between hyperactivity in children and certain food colors, additives, and even natural substances in foods. Dr. Ben Feingold has suggested that a direct association exists between these synthetic food colors and flavors and the clinical syndrome vaguely defined as hyperkinesis or hyperactivity in young children. This is frequently associated with lack of attention span and significant disruption of family, and school, as well as learning disabilities. Although many investigators question whether such a syndrome really exists, such a diagnosis has been established in our society, although it may very well be a social diagnosis established for controlling children in schools.

*Is "Hyperactivity" a Social Category*

However, a fair number of clinical and many testimonial reports claim that a certain percentage of children with this syndrome, somewhere between 30 and 50 percent, improve markedly when placed on an elimination diet from which all additives as well as certain natural foods alleged to contain salicylates are eliminated. Unfortunately there is not yet clear-cut scientific evidence proving that the removal of these additives in elimination diets is the *cause* of the improvement in these children, although such studies are under way.

*Love, Warmth, and Care Cofactors in Cure?*

However, I must emphasize that many families have experienced significant, virtually miraculous improvement in their children when they have been placed on such a diet. Whether these changes can be attributed to a general improvement of nutritional status, or a change in the sociocultural milieu of the family, or whether they are truly due to the removal of certain of these toxins from individuals who are particularly susceptible to them, is unknown. Whatever the cause of this improvement might be, the fact that it occurs is something that must be accepted, and certainly even though the responses may not be quite as dramatic as those seen when drugs such as Ritalin are administered, dietary change is much safer, and the long-term potential effects, instead of being harmful as might be expected with drug therapy, can only be considered as beneficial.

*If Tom Sawyer Lived, Would He Be Declared Hyperactive?*

SCHIZOPHRENIA   Acute schizophrenia and other forms of mental illness are not permanent, but are acute illnesses, usually responding to many types of therapy, primarily release of stress, and generally with a good prognosis, although obviously with the tendency for recurrence when the conditions of stress recur for that given individual. In fact, the entire concept of the nature and meaning of mental illness is undergoing rapid change, and some psychiatrists go so far as to question whether there is any such thing or whether mental illnesses are merely alterations in behavior under conditions of stress—defense mechanisms to avoid more serious types of breakdowns.

The term *orthomolecular medicine* was coined by the eminent Nobel laureate Dr. Linus Pauling in 1968, to describe "the right molecules in the right amounts." Varying the concentration of the molecules normally present in the human body, Dr. Pauling believes, will prevent and treat disease more effectively than synthetic drugs.

It has long been known that a deficiency in virtually any of the vitamins would lead to alterations in behavior or mental state. Classic examples of these have been deficiency of vitamin $B_1$, or thiamine, leading to the disease known as beriberi, and the psychotic episodes occurring in deficiencies of nicotinic acid in the disease known as pellagra. Dr. Pauling believed that because of the tremendous variability in the human population, a considerable number of people might be suffering from deficiencies of certain nutrients leading to diseases because these individuals have much higher requirements than the majority of the population. In fact, even prior to Dr. Pauling's becoming interested in this area, other workers in the field had postulated similar theories.

*Certain Vitamins and Minerals Increase Rate of Remission*

Orthomolecular psychiatrists, such as Dr. David Hawkins of the North Nassau Mental Health Clinic in New York, inform us that 80 percent of acute schizophrenics who receive vitamin/ mineral supplementation, in addition to the normal regimen of phenothiazine, are released and not rehospitalized. This compares with a success rate of 35 to 45 percent for acute schizophrenics treated only with the drug. The vitamin-treated group often discontinue the drug without problems.

The amounts given these patients vary, being different for individual schizophrenics, but generally range between 4 to 8 grams of vitamin C, about 8 to 20 grams of niacin or niacinamide, about 400 to 800 mg of pyridoxine, and often 400 to 800 units of vitamin E, as well as the same amount of thiamine, all on a daily basis. Zinc is the most significant mineral in this regimen, and also varies with individual needs.

*Cures May Be Related to Placebo Effect*

Many other types of mental illness have also been attributed to and allegedly cured by readjustment of the dose level of various nutrients. But attempts to carry out carefully controlled studies of the effectiveness of the orthomolecular regimen often seem to be related to the bias of the investigator, so that at present it is quite impossible to state with any degree of certainty whether or not the orthomolecular approach is effective. Never-theless, the therapies outlined by the orthomolecular psychia-trists are generally quite harmless, and certainly if an individual suffering from some mental illness, particularly one as serious as schizophrenia, shows definite benefits from the orthomolecu-lar regimen, it must not be discounted.

However, my anxiety in this area arises from the promise of a magical cure, and it is against such promises that I must warn the reader who may have friends or relatives suffering from schizophrenia. A fair number of controlled studies have shown that the effects of these vitamins and minerals on schizo-phrenics are no greater than placebos. Therefore we must ap-proach the entire problem of orthomolecular medicine and psychiatry with great caution at this time, and realize that it is a highly controversial field and not one that has been solidly demonstrated to have the degree of effectiveness that the enthu-siasts would lead us to believe. Nevertheless, where there is success with the vitamins and minerals, and patients are able to be weaned from liver-damaging tranquilizers, I wholeheart-edly support the results.

# Viral Diseases (Colds, Hepatitis, Influenza, Mononucleosis, Pneumonia)

These illnesses are all treated with massive doses of vitamin C by Dr. William Cathcart III of Incline Village, Nevada. Based on seven thousand cases, Dr. Cathcart believes that this approach is the most effective and safest of all those available. Where he used to hospitalize many people for some of these illnesses, he now tells them to take vitamin C in the granule form, at home, on a megadose level—apparently with very satisfactory results. The following article, authored by Linus Pauling (1978), describes the work of this orthomolecular physi-cian, including dosage instructions given his patients.

*7,000 Patients Aided by Vitamin C*

### Viral Diseases and Vitamin C
#### BY LINUS PAULING

Dr. B. J. Luberoff, editor of the journal, *Chemtech,* which is published by the American Chemical Society, interviewed Dr. Cathcart recently (*Chemtech,* Feb. 1978), questioning him especially about his use of vitamin C in his medical practice. In 1971, while he was still practicing orthopedic surgery in San Mateo, Dr. Cathcart read my book, "Vitamin C and the Common Cold," and tried taking a few grams of vitamin C at the onset of a cold in order to check whether or not it would stop the cold. He then wrote me that two grams of vitamin C every hour seemed to do the job, but that he preferred taking eight grams at one time, and that this was usually effective.

In his interview he said, "After reading Pauling and everything else I could on the subject, I started 'experimenting' with vitamin C, first on myself and the family, and then on a few selected patients. In San Mateo I had little opportunity to treat patients with vitamin C. Besides, as an orthopedic surgeon, I seldom saw patients who had colds, or other viral diseases. So I commuted to Incline Village every week for a year. . . . where I went into association with a general practitioner who planned to go to another town after about another year. During that year I demonstrated that, properly used, vitamin C could decrease most of the morbidity and all of the mortality from viral diseases. I contacted Pauling about this, and he said that he knew of no other physician who was doing exactly what I was doing."

Dr. Cathcart then said that Dr. Fred Klenner of Reidsville, North Carolina, had during the past thirty years found that he could detoxify most virus diseases with intravenous doses of vitamin C, which he uses even for carbon monoxide poisoning, barbiturate poisoning, and snake bites.

What Dr. Cathcart discovered was that, although most people develop a mild diarrhea when they take 10 or 15 grams of vitamin C in divided doses in one day when they are well, they can tolerate much higher amounts if they are ill.

He stated, "The astonishing thing is that the same person—the patient who when well gets diarrhea on, say, 12 grams—when ill with a moderate cold can take 30 to 60 grams, sometimes even 150 grams, and with viral diseases such as mononucleosis or viral pneumonia I've used in excess of 200 grams a day without its producing diarrhea. . . . In some cases the body evidently *needs* that much, albeit for only a short time. With mononucleosis or viral pneumonias, during the first couple of days of the disease we sometimes see a need for that half pound of the vitamin. . . . Essentially, the sicker you are, the more you can take, and taking enough—*and that's important*—seems to detoxify you. You get well quickly. And as you do, you find that you can tolerate less and less ascorbic acid until you go back to normal when you are well."

Dr. Cathcart pointed out that it is known that vitamin C has many functions in the body, including its involvement in several enzyme-catalyzed reactions and in the body's ability to make colagen, dentyne, adrenaline, and corticosteroids. It maintains proper functioning of the immune system, the blood coagulation system, and controls the metabolism of several amino acids.

With respect to the treatment of patients, he said, "My practice is to let the body take as much vitamin C as it needs . . . to take an amount proportional to the amount of toxin that's around. Remember, everyone else has been talking about a fixed dose, usually at what I consider to be only a homeopathic level. Those studies go from two or maybe four grams a day and they see little clinical effect and no effect statistically. That doesn't surprise me. If you have a 100-gram cold . . . it's my custom to put a number before the name of a disease to represent the amount of vitamin C that the patient can consume the first couple of days of the disease without diarrhea . . . so that if you have a 100-gram cold and the patient is taking roughly 100 grams a day, you will quickly eliminate perhaps 90% of the symptoms of the disease. But if you treat that same cold with 2 grams or even 20 grams a day, you won't see much happen.

"In some cases, especially if treated early, it almost seems as if megadoses were killing viruses. With bad colds or influenza we don't seem to shorten the duration of the infection, but we render patients sufficiently asymptomatic so that they weather the infection without complications. Most of the time my patients don't have to miss any work time. If you're using enough ascorbic acid it will promptly take a fever down to normal, and you won't have the normal aches and pains of flu-like diseases. . . . The typical patient who get mononucleosis is exactly the one who does the best on vitamin C: older teenagers or young adults are just fantastic vitamin-C takers. They can understand the bowel tolerance idea, have iron stomachs, and couldn't care less about slight gas and diarrhea when they have this horrible disease. In fact, the sicker a patient is the better he does because the relief of symptoms is so dramatic that they don't need any arguments to convince them to continue treatment. So what usually happens is that in three to five days the symptoms are 90% relieved. . . . The important thing with mono or other responsive diseases is that we can get people back to work in days.

"The other disease that is very specific is infectious hepatitis. . . . It's a cinch for vitamin C. The difference between the course of the disease with and without vitamin C is quite obvious if only because hepatitis is a disease that we can put numbers on. There are various enzyme systems that we can follow to show the course of the disease. Infectious hepatitis can be mild, where the patient is just a little yellow and maybe a bit tender in the abdomen, but not very sick. But the patients I'm talking about—20 of them, at least—were profoundly ill with hepatitis, and here again we were able to detoxify them in three to five days. It generally took about six days for the jaundice to clear. In two or three days the urine returned to normal color.

"Hepatitis is a serious problem following blood transfusions. As a matter of fact the whole system of gathering blood in this country is undergoing revision because people who sell their blood have a high incidence of hepatitis. That's why they're trying to go completely to a voluntary system. I'm not sure that's necessary because it's apparently so simple to control hepatitis: just give patients vitamin C after blood transfusions. One Japanese physician (Dr. Fukumi Miroshige, Non-resident Fellow of the Linus Pauling Institute) has shown that his patients don't get hepatitis if he puts them on maintenance doses of ascorbic acid following blood transfusions. Anybody who is stressed enough to need a blood transfusion should be getting large doses of vitamin C anyway."

Dr. Cathcart talked about side effects of large doses of vitamin C, saying that they seem not to be very important. When asked about kidney stones, he answered, "I've never seen an oxalate kidney stone among my regular vitamin C takers. There is a theory that says that ascorbic acid breaks down to oxalate so that if a person had difficulty handling oxalate, he could precipitate oxalate stones. But the situation is paradoxical: I'll grant that if a person did have difficulty handling oxalates, he might increase his oxalate load, but the paradox is that if a person takes vitamin C in large doses, as large as I've been talking about, it somehow makes the oxalate more soluble in the urine. Anyway, the pragmatic fact is that in my experience oxalate stones caused by vitamin C are not something to worry about."

Dr. Cathcart, who has now been practicing in Incline Village for seven years, stated that he had given megadoses of vitamin C to about 7000 patients. He said that the manufacturers of vitamin C think that Incline Village consumes more vitamin C per capita than any other place in the world. When asked about danger, he said, "If a patient who's accustomed to high vitamin C intake is hospitalized or otherwise comes under the care of certain physicians, the physician may cut off the C . . . and do it just when the patient needs it most."

When asked about vitamin C and the common cold, he said, "I think that a person who has no really good reason to take vitamin C, no immediate illness, probably should do as Pauling says and take somewhere around 4 grams a day. People with allergies may find that they are more comfortable with higher amounts. I'm the last person in the world to maintain that you will never get a cold if you're taking maintenance doses of vitamin C. I get occasional colds, but I can block the symptoms with vitamin C. I never cease to be amazed at the number of patients who report to me that they used to get colds all the time and never get them since they began taking vitamin C. . . . I take 10 to 15 grams a day, first because I used to have hay fever—vitamin C takes care of hay fever nicely in about two-thirds of all cases—and second, because there is evidence that it reduces cholesterol and thus helps prevent arteriosclerosis. Third, I believe that vitamin C contributes to prevention of some cancers."

When asked about the basis for his statement about cancer, Dr. Cathcart referred to the work done in Scotland by Dr. Ewan Cameron, a Non-resident Fellow of the Linus Pauling Institute, and he concluded by saying, "I think that anyone with cancer should be taking high doses of vitamin C."

## The Limitations of Nutritional Therapy

Being a therapy in its infancy, there is a tendency for all therapeutic ideas regarding food and diet to appear equally reasonable or unreasonable, depending on one's degree of desperation. And so people turn to their doctors, "healers," chiropractors, dentists, yoga teachers, for some sort of dietary salvation.

It is tempting for both client and healer to go beyond the agreed-upon realm of competence, delving into areas not within the scope of nutritional therapy nor the ken of training of most nutritional counselors.

Many people come to nutritionists hoping to find a fundamentally diet-related cause/cure for their distress, which is often more a reflection of the vicissitudes of existence than the result of diet per se. Yes, diet and vitamin approaches will help somewhat, but to expect the nutritionist to eliminate all inner disharmonies with the dietary equivalent of the "magic bullet" of Fleming is both unrealistic and potentially dangerous, both for client and nutritionist.

So many dietary theories have attracted cult followings (including the cult of overeating, an American contribution) and been found to "cure" various disease states, mainly due to the placebo effect. If a person who is not too ill has faith in her "adviser" and follows the dietary rules like a good though frightened child, about 80 percent of all patients will get better, about the same number who improve on placebos. And so we must not underestimate the mother of all medicines, the placebo, when evaluating the claims of our dietary messiahs.

Nevertheless, it is worthwhile to look at a few disorders and associated nutritional approaches. While some of the food prescriptions and proscriptions and supplements used are based on anecdotal material, good, solid references can be found to substantiate these regimens, particularly in Rogers (1957), Shive (1957), Williams (1973), Fredericks (1965, 1969), Jarvis (1960), Rudolph (1977), and Miller (1977).

## Nutri-Treatment of Selected Disorders*

Here I include some disorders and the nutritional approaches suggested by several leading researchers and clinicians. Being "experimental" in the sense that any newer therapy is doubted until proven efficacious by million-dollar experi-

* All references to medicinal plants are taken from *Weiner's Herbal* (1980), where more detailed references are listed. Dosages of various supplements are omitted owing to individual differences that can only be approximated following appropriate laboratory work (hair, urine, serum analysis). This brief chart is *not* to be used for diagnostic or prescriptive purposes; it is compiled for the utility of physicians and patients working *together*.

# Nutri-Treatment of Selected Disorders (for review purposes only)

| Disorder | Foods to Eat | Foods to Avoid | Supplements |
|---|---|---|---|
| Alcoholism | Protein; complex carbohydrates | Refined carbohydrates (especially sugars, honey) | Multivitamin/mineral formula; niacinamide; glutamine (1–4 grams daily) |
| Arthritis (rheumatoid) | Low protein (fish okay); high complex carbohydrates (vegetables), 6 meals daily; juniper berry tea; apple cider vinegar (2 tsp) + honey (2 tsp), in glass of water | Animal proteins (milk, eggs, meat, poultry) | Niacinamide (400 mg–2,250 mg daily); pantothenic acid; pyridoxine; vitamins A, C, D, E, B-complex; copper; cobalt, magnesium, manganese, phosphorus (and rub on wheat germ oil) |
| Cataracts (in diabetes mellitus) | Fruits and vegetables (particularly the skin, peel, and outer layers of citrus) | | Bioflavonoids |
| Colds | | | Vitamin C 3–10 grams daily |
| Constipation | Fiber-rich foods (fruits and vegetables, whole grains); rhubarb tea | Black tea; all tannin-rich foods and drinks | |
| Diabetes | Refined carbohydrates; animal fats | | Vitamin A, $B_2$, E; chromium, manganese, potassium, zinc, magnesium |
| Epilepsy | Mugwort tea | Caffeine; sweets | Vitamin $B_{12}$ |
| Gallbladder | Emphasize raw or steamed vegetables, ripe fruits; limit starches; lean meat; olive oil on salads | Fatty food; fried foods; sweets; butter | |
| Gout | Emphasize vegetables; fruits; cereals; milk, cheese, eggs; nuts; juniper berry and pennyroyal tea | Organ meats; anchovies; sardines; shellfish; spinach; bran | Vitamin C, B-complex |
| Herpes Simplex | | | Lysine; zinc; vitamin C |
| High Blood Pressure | Potassium-rich foods (bananas, potatoes) | Salt and hidden salt (i.e., cheese, bread, pickles, olives, sauces, etc.); no fried foods; reduce alcohol | *Cadmium* must be eliminated |

| Ailment | Diet/Foods | Avoid | Supplements |
|---|---|---|---|
| Impotence | Whole foods; milk; honey; ginseng | Preserved foods (especially with nitrates and nitrites) | Multivitamin/minerals; extra zinc; vitamin E |
| Insomnia | Passionflower or valerian tea | Caffeine; late meals; heavy meals | Vitamin C, E, B-complex; calcium/magnesium |
| Kidney Ailments | Vegetables emphasized; shave grass tea | High animal-protein diet limited; limit sweets and refined carbohydrates | Minimal supplementation |
| Kidney Stones | Cranberry juice; drink 2 quarts pure water daily | | |
| Calcium phosphate stones | | Cheese; milk; alkalis; vitamin D | Aluminum hydroxide gel |
| Calcium oxalate stones | | Oxalic acids (rhubarb, spinach, cocoa, chocolate, wheat germ) | Magnesium oxide; vitamin $B_6$ |
| Lead Toxicity | High-protein, high-sulfur diet (natural chelation) | | B-complex (especially niacin); choline |
| Migraine | High protein; fresh fruits and vegetables | All sweets | B-complex; vitamin E; calcium/magnesium; potassium; manganese |
| Nervousness | Passionflower tea; simple diet | Coffee, tea; spicy foods | Laxative (magnesium oxide); witch hazel in bath water; club moss sprinkled on |
| Rashes (or hives) | Bland diet | Unripe fruits; fatty meats; crab; fish; oysters; pickles | Calcium/magnesium in balance |
| Rheumatism (also see Arthritis) | Devil's-claw tea | | |
| Seasickness | Eat sparingly of dry foods; sprinkle on cayenne pepper | Liquids | Biotin (150–300 µg daily) |
| Seborrhea | Yeast; liver; rice bran; soybeans; nuts | Egg white (and mayonnaise, etc.) | Vitamin A; B-complex; sulfur; biotin |
| Skin Problems (eczema, dermatitis, psoriasis) | Comfrey tea; yarrow tea; simplify diet | All spicy foods; all fried foods | Vitamins A, C, D, B-complex; lysine; zinc; copper; molybdenum |
| Tooth Decay | Lactobacilli; whole foods | Refined carbohydrates; reduced oxalates (spinach); limit juices | |
| Urinary Tract Infections | Spotted wintergreen tea; yogurt | | Zinc; magnesium |

ments, these treatments are nevertheless the best leads we have for ailments that continue to plague allopathic medicine. (In some cases, of course, such as with gout, even the most cynical physician will agree that abstaining from purine-rich foods will affect the disorder positively.)

## The Acid-Base Question

Health-food literature frequently refers to the acid-base balance within, suggesting foods that will move the pH in either direction. Just as various plants have differing needs for soil (acid, neutral, alkaline), so too do we. And here is where the lists of acid-producing foods countered by the alkaline foods come in handily. Before reviewing these lists, we must ask if this acid-base idea is valid.

To answer the question indirectly I include a recent article about a genetic disorder that destroys the acid-base balance. Following is the dietary treatment. Written by Winifred Cox, and first appearing in the University of California *Clip Sheet* (April 29, 1980), this information should disarm the most skeptical reader who thinks all health-food literature deficient of scientific validity.

## Genetic Disease Treated with Diet

After seven months of treatment, Matthew's physicians at the University of California, San Diego Hospital are willing to predict that he will survive a genetic disease that has killed or severely retarded most of its other victims.

And there are indications that Matthew's intellectual development may be able to catch up with his remarkable physical progress.

At one month of age, Matthew was diagnosed as having methylmalonic acidemia. His body cannot convert the protein he eats into energy. Instead, several amino acids in that protein are converted into a toxic side-product, methylmalonic acid, which destroys the delicate acid-base balance of his body, and poisons his system.

Almost since birth, this acid-overload has caused twenty-month-old Matthew a host of problems—from dehydration and severe rashes, to an almost complete arrest of his mental and physical development. On several occasions Matthew has become comatose, and neared death.

At thirteen months of age, Matthew was brought to UCSD, to the care of metabolic specialists, William Nyhan and Drew Kelts. Eleven years ago Nyhan saved the life of another infant, Loren, one of the few children known to have survived this rare disease.

## The Missing Enzyme

Neither Matthew nor Loren responds to vitamin B-12 treatments, which some methylmalonic acidemia children respond to. Apparently, these two youngsters have normal B-12 levels, but are deficient in a partner enzyme, called methylmalonyl-Co-A-isomerase. Both substances must be present in order to convert amino acids the children take in through food into energy. Unfortunately, there is no substitute for methylmalonyl-Co-A-isomerase, the missing enzyme.

Nyhan had to devise an entirely new approach to Loren's treatment—to somehow restrict her intake of protein and amino acids to the precise amount her body could handle. That plan worked for Loren, and has also been the basis of Matthew's care.

Because the amino acids that these youngsters cannot handle—isoleucine and valine—are in all protein foods, their diet had to be constructed from its chemical components. Matthew receives continual, intravenous feedings of a synthetic protein-fat-carbohydrate formula. The amino acids in that formula are synthesized in Japan, and then combined in a metabolic laboratory at the University of California, Los Angeles. Carbohydrates, fats, and "safe" amino acids and proteins are supplied by another synthetic formula prepared by UCSD dieticians.

Samples of Matthew's blood and urine are routinely taken, to determine if excess methylmalonic acid is accumulating. When it does, Matthew's diet is immediately reformulated to lower its isoleucine and valine content.

Matthew's diet is the most critical aspect of his round-the-clock regime of physical therapy, speech training and intensive nursing care. His treatment is administered in UCSD's General Clinical Research Center—a unit equipped and staffed to handle extremely complex and experimental treatment programs.

## Better Prognosis

Now, at twenty months, Matthew is a chubby 24 pounds. It was apparent, upon admittance, that his physical and mental development had stopped at three months of age. After treatment, his physical development has advanced to a nine-month level, and his intellectual development has gained at least six months.

The remarkable developmental spurt made by Loren, who, despite an entire year in which her brain stopped developing, attained normal intelligence by the age of 13, gives Matthew's physicians hope for his continued mental development.

Besides the reward of saving a youngster's life, supervising Matthew's case has had other payoffs for the UC San Diego physicians.

"Since many metabolic diseases stem from a missing or inactive enzyme, a variation of Matthew's diet may work for other children with metabolic defects," Dr. Kelts says.

"Matthew's treatment should also tell us what is the minimum amount of protein children must have to meet their growth needs. It's impossible to determine this from normal children since whatever amino acids they don't use for growth, they convert into energy," says Kelts.

One group of nutritionists states that a "balanced diet contains 40% acid-forming foods and 60% alkaline." In the following chart note that beef, poultry, fish, and egg yolk are acid-forming foods, while alcohol, caffeine, rice, soy, pasta, sugar, tobacco, and wheat are "*highly* acid." To balance these common dietary components it would be wise to include more alkaline foods, and especially those noted as "highly alkaline" (bean sprouts, dates, figs, prunes, sour grapes, and Swiss chard). Teas such as clover, sage, mint, strawberry, and alfalfa are a wiser choice, in this light, than is coffee, an acid-producing food. Garlic, onions, spinach, tomatoes, and eggplant—all commonly associated with Italian food—are also alkaline, balancing well

## The Acid-Alkaline Chart

| Acid | Highly Acid | Neutral |
| --- | --- | --- |
| Beans (kidney, navy, white, garbanzo) | Alcohol | OILS: |
| | Artichoke | Avocado |
| Beef | Barley | Olive |
| Blueberries | Bread | Sesame |
| Brussels sprouts | Buckwheat | Coconut |
| Cashews | Caffeine | Soy |
| Coconut, dried | Corn, dry yellow | Sunflower |
| Cranberries | Custards | Safflower |
| Egg yolk | Drugs | Cottonseed |
| Filberts | Flours (all) | Almond |
| Fish | Ginger, preserved | Linseed |
| Fruit (dried, sulfured, canned, sugared, jams, jellies) | Honey | FATS: |
| | Lentils, dry | Butter |
| | Maté | Cream |
| Gelatin | Millet | Margarine |
| Goat, meat and dairy | Oatmeal | Animal fat |
| Grapes, sweet | Peanuts | Lard |
| Milk products, pasteurized | Potato, sweet | |
| Mushrooms | Rice (all) | |
| Mutton | Rye grain | |
| Pecans | Sorghum | |
| Plums, Damson | Soy, bread and noodles | |
| Pork | Spaghetti products | |
| Poultry | Squash, except winter | |
| Sorghum grain | Sugar, cane and raw | |
| Water chestnuts | Tobacco | |
| | Walnuts, English | |
| | Wheat grain | |

## *The Acid-Alkaline Chart (Cont.)*

| Alkaline | High Alkaline | Highly Alkaline |
| --- | --- | --- |
| Agar | Almonds | Beans, dried lima, string |
| Alfalfa | Avocado | Bean sprouts |
| Apple and cider | Banana, speckled only | Currants |
| Apricot, fresh | Beans, fresh lima | Dandelion greens |
| Artichokes, globe | Beet | Dates |
| Asparagus | Blackberries | Figs, especially black |
| Bamboo shoots | Carrot | Prunes |
| Beans, snap | Chives | Swiss chard |
| Berries, most | Cranberries | |
| Bok choy | Endive | |
| Broccoli | Grapes, sour | |
| Cabbage (red, white, savoy, | Kale | |
| Chinese) | Peach, dried | |
| Cantaloupe | Persimmon | |
| Cauliflower | Plum | |
| Celery | Pomegranate | |
| Cherries | Raspberries | |
| Chestnuts | Spinach | |
| Chicory | | |
| Coconut, fresh meat and | | |
| milk | | |
| Coffee substitutes | | |
| Collards | | |
| Corn, fresh sweet | | |
| Daikon | | |
| Eggplant | | |
| Escarole | | |
| Garlic | | |
| Ginger, dry | | |
| Gooseberries | | |
| Guava | | |
| Horseradish, fresh raw | | |
| Kelp | | |
| Kohlrabi | | |
| Leek | | |
| Lemon and peel | | |
| Lettuce | | |
| Lime | | |
| Loganberries | | |
| Mango | | |
| Melons | | |
| Milk (raw, whey, yogurt, | | |
| acidophilus) | | |
| Nectarine | | |
| Okra | | |
| Olives, sun-dried | | |
| Onion | | |
| Orange | | |
| Papaya | | |
| Parsley | | |
| Parsnip | | |
| Peach, fresh | | |
| Pear, fresh | | |

## The Acid-Alkaline Chart (Cont.)

| Alkaline | High Alkaline | Highly Alkaline |
|---|---|---|
| Peas | | |
| Pepper, green and red | | |
| Pineapple, ripe | | |
| Potato, except sweet | | |
| Prickly pear | | |
| Pumpkin | | |
| Quince | | |
| Radishes | | |
| Rhubarb | | |
| Sapodilla | | |
| Sauerkraut, lemon | | |
| Squash, winter | | |
| Tamari | | |
| Tangerine | | |
| Teas (clover, sage, mint, strawberry, alfalfa) | | |
| Tomato | | |
| Turnip | | |
| Watercress | | |
| Yeast | | |

Developed by Anabolic Foods, Irvine, California.

with meats, which are acid foods. This example of wise ethnic dietetics can be applied to other cuisines simply by listing the foods in a typical dish, referring to the chart, and noting their acid-alkaline scores.

Having looked at the "food as medicine" question, we are now ready to see the dietary interrelationships in one of our most dreaded scourges: cancer.

# 11 DIET AND CANCER

Statistical "facts" garnered from the research literature abound. Such facts by themselves are of little value; what is required is a point of view generated by an interpreter of these facts. Most competent writers can present reputable scientific studies to support both sides of a nutritional issue. Vitamin C, for example, can be shown as being effective, ineffective, or harmful for each of a wide variety of complaints. My point of view, based upon personal experience, observations of cases from my clinical practice, and hard epidemiological studies of whole populations lead me to support the usage of vitamin C for treating disorders such as colds, mononucleosis, pneumonia, hepatitis, and certain types of cancer.

An excellent volume on the subject by Dr. Linus Pauling has recently appeared (Cameron and Pauling, 1979). Just as Thomas Henry Huxley was known as "Darwin's bulldog," it would be a great honor if I were to be known as "Pauling's bulldog," because, in evaluating the evidence for myself, I am convinced that the man is fifty to one hundred years ahead of his nearest competitors in terms of breakthrough biochemical thinking.

*Vitamin C Useful to Prevent Some Cancers*

It seems that only pedestrian research is funded by the Nutrition and Cancer Division of the National Cancer Institute. People of Dr. Pauling's league, or Dr. Albert Szent-Gyorgyi's, are almost automatically screened out of the vast federal budget devoted to this question.

*Pedestrian Research Too Often Funded*

An example of the bias against Dr. Pauling—an unscientific bias at that—is clearly presented in a critique of *Vitamin C and Cancer* done by the reputable Mayo Clinic. It seems that when it comes to Dr. Pauling, even a clinic of such repute is unable to overcome the bias of investigators within that institution. The following article first appeared in the newsletter of the Linus Pauling Institute of Science and Medicine, Vol. 1, #7, Fall 1979; it is reprinted in its entirety to enable the reader to draw his own conclusions about the possible effectiveness of this vitamin against cancer.

## The Mayo Clinic Trial of Vitamin C and Cancer

During the last year a controlled clinical trial of the value of vitamin C in the treatment of patients with advanced cancer was carried out under the direction of Dr. Charles G. Moertel, in the Division of Medical Oncology and the Cancer Statistics Unit, Mayo Clinic, Rochester, Minnesota, with the support in part of a contract with the National Institutes of Health. The results of this trial have been misrepresented in newspaper articles, which have stated, for example, that Dr. Cameron and Dr. Pauling were wrong in claiming benefit for patients treated with vitamin C, and were even misrepresented in *The New England Journal of Medicine.*

The trial was carried out because of the continued efforts of Dr. Cameron and Dr. Pauling to have the National Cancer Institute investigate this question. In 1973 Dr. Pauling went to the National Cancer Institute, in Bethesda, Maryland, in order to show officials the case histories of the first 40 patients with advanced cancer treated by Dr. Cameron with high doses of vitamin C as their only therapy, and to ask that the National Cancer Institute carry out or sponsor a double-blind randomized controlled trial, in order to check the promising observations made in Vale of Leven Hospital. The officials of the National Cancer Institute refused to carry out such a trial, however, and repeated their refusal for several years during which Dr. Pauling continued his efforts. Finally, in 1977, after he had again visited Bethesda and had urged Dr. Vincent DeVita, Chief of the Clinical Trials Section of the National Cancer Institute, to arrange for such a controlled trial and had been turned down, he wrote a very strong letter to Dr. DeVita. Dr. DeVita replied that he would see if he could arrange for a controlled trial to be made, and later he informed Dr. Pauling that Dr. Moertel of the Mayo Clinic had agreed to carry it out.

*Chemotherapy Can Destroy the Immune System*    When the study was being planned Dr. Moertel wrote to Dr. Pauling that he wanted to repeat the Vale of Leven trial as closely as possible. Dr. Pauling then wrote him that to do so would require that his terminal cancer patients not have received heavy doses of cytotoxic chemotherapy, because this chemotherapy damages the immune system and may prevent the vitamin C from being effective. The following sentences are from Dr. Pauling's letter of 9 August 1978 to Dr. Moertel:

*"In my last letter to you I pointed out to you that the patients studied by Dr. Cameron had not received chemotherapy. The cytotoxic drugs damage the body's protective mechanisms, and vitamin C probably functions largely by potentiating these mechanisms. Accordingly, if you hope, as you stated in your letter, to repeat the work of Cameron as closely as possible, you should be careful to use only patients who have*

*not received chemotherapy. . . . On page 2 (of your letter) there is no mention of earlier chemotherapeutic treatment as a contraindication for patient eligibility. I think that this question might be important, however, and I recommend that you be sure that there are a sufficient number of patients enrolled who have not received chemotherapy. Otherwise the trial cannot be described as repeating the work of Cameron."*

In fact, when the paper on the Mayo Clinic trial was published [Creagan, E. T.; Moertel, C. G.; et al., "Failure of high-dose vitamin C (ascorbic acid) therapy to benefit patients with advanced cancer," *New England J. of Medicine,* September 27, 1979] it was seen that Dr. Moertel had ignored this advice. The authors state that 50 of the 100 ascorbate-treated patients in the Vale of Leven study had received chemotherapy and high-energy radiation, whereas in fact only 4 had received chemotherapy and only 20 had received high energy radiation. The failure of the investigators to observe a large effect of vitamin C in the patients shows, as Dr. Cameron and Dr. Pauling predicted, that the value of vitamin C is much less for patients whose immune systems have been damaged by chemotherapy than for those who have not received chemotherapy.

*Dr. Pauling's Careful Study Not Duplicated Accurately by Detractors*

The Mayo Clinic study seems to have answered an important question. Dr. Cameron and Dr. Pauling have pointed out that chemotherapy badly damages the body's natural protective mechanisms, especially the immune system, and that, inasmuch as vitamin C is effective against cancer largely by potentiating these mechanisms, patients who have been treated with chemotherapy probably would not respond well to treatment with vitamin C, but Dr. Cameron and Dr. Pauling did not have reliable information as to how great this effect would be. The Mayo Clinic study seems to show that patients who have received treatment with chemotherapy respond very poorly to subsequent vitamin C therapy. Adults with solid tumors in Scotland usually are not treated with chemotherapy because experience has shown that the benefit is small. On the other hand, the benefit of treatment with vitamin C is large, having the important advantages that it is inexpensive and that it increases the patient's sense of well-being, permitting him usually to lead a good life.

Dr. Cameron and Dr. Pauling have urged the National Cancer Institute to sponsor another controlled trial, with patients with advanced cancer who have not received treatment with cytotoxic chemotherapeutic agents, but it is still uncertain as to whether this trial will be carried out.

# How Vitamin C Works

Dr. Albert Szent-Gyorgyi received a Nobel Prize in Medicine in 1937 for his discovery of vitamin C, and in 1954 he was awarded the Albert Lasker Prize for his theory of muscle contraction. He is also the codiscoverer of the citric acid cycle,

*Ascorbic Acid Promotes Normal Cell Division*

a fundamental mechanism of human metabolism, also known as the Krebs cycle. Dr. Szent-Gyorgyi granted an exclusive interview to the editors of *Nutrition Today,* which resulted in a series of imaginative drawings on how vitamin C might work at the cellular level. According to this article in the September–October 1979 issue of *Nutrition Today,* ascorbic acid promotes normal cell division, not the type of cell division that creates half-divided, half-united cells that go berserk and become cancerous. This eighty-seven-year-old scientist believes that vitamin C ends up in our cells, creating furious electron exchanges that are responsible for a stability that is otherwise impossible to achieve. He speculates, "Maybe the substance, ascorbic acid, is not a vitamin, but life's most important chemical." In attempting to describe the activity of ascorbic acid at the atomic level, Szent-Gyorgyi contends that most of our body's protein molecules and their atoms are dormant in the body because they are in a harmonious electronic balance. To activate their life force, they must be "desaturated," and this is done by removing the electron. Vitamin C in the ascorbate form has an affinity for oxygen, and since there is oxygen in each cell, the stage is set for truly amazing activity. Ascorbate releases an electron to oxygen and becomes a free radical available to receive electrons from other sources; in this case, an electron is donated by methyl glyoxal. This substance is derived from the enzyme glyoxalase, and so when ascorbate gives up an electron to oxygen and becomes a free radical and receives an electron from methyl glyoxal in cellular protein, the protein is desaturated and comes to life, the beginning of all fundamental activity. This "bioelectronic theory of life" holds that "the degree of electron saturation and desaturation determines whether the cell remains or divides abnormally and becomes cancerous."

This is not to argue that vitamin C is a cancer cure. However, being intricately involved at the most fundamental cellular level, it is highly likely that ascorbic acid is certainly one of our most essential nutrients.

# Chlorophyll: An Essential Anticancer Agent

*Wheat Grass*
*Juice*
*Chlorophyll*
*Rich*

Work with other substances tends to support Dr. Szent-Gyorgyi's theory. For example, in an article by Chiu-Nan Lai entitled "Chlorophyll: The Active Factor in Wheat Sprout Extract Inhibiting the Metabolic Activation of Carcinogens in

Vitro," we learn that this fundamental green plant substance is the major active factor in wheat sprouts which causes the inhibition of mutagenic effects of carcinogens. Like vitamin C, chlorophyll is capable of electron transfer in the absence of light. Structurally it is much different from ascorbic acid, being similar to heme, which is a porphyrin structure with magnesium in the center with a hydrophobic tail. While chlorophyll is unlike other inhibitors of carcinogenesis on a structural level, such as vitamin A analogs, selenium, BHT, vitamin E, and others, many of these substances share the chemical similarities of "antioxidants"; further, "the redox potentials of chlorophyll have been reported to be in the range of 0.64–0.78 volt against a standard hydrogen electrode for the reaction shown below:

$$Ch^+ + e^- \longrightarrow Ch$$

This is in the same range as that reported for vitamin A analogs and selenium."

The author suggests that chlorophyll acts as an antioxidant in the Ames bacteria test, where the mutagenic effect of carcinogens was tried. It is interesting that wheat grass juice, a popular item in health-food stores, shows such activity, but this is not a totally unexpected finding. As far back as 1940 chlorophyll was reported to be clinically useful for treating infections and suppurative diseases by Gruskin (1940), who learned "that it has never been shown to be toxic in therapeutic doses, and its potential as a nontoxic chemopreventive agent appears promising." Of course, many vegetables that have been screened in this bacteria test have been found to have antimutagenic activity, and so, acting on an atomic level the way ascorbate does, by transferring electrons, chlorophyll from green vegetables is a wise dietary component.

# Nutrition and the Immune System

At the level of the immune system, where much frantic work in cancer is being directed today, Dr. D. F. Horrobin has advanced one of the most interesting theories in an article entitled, "The Nutritional Regulation of T-Lymphocyte Function." According to this hypothesis most diseases that we do not yet understand seem to be related to T-lymphocyte abnormalities—diseases such as abnormal susceptibility to infections, autoimmune disorders of different types, cancer, rheumatoid arthritis, multiple sclerosis, Crohn's disease, primary biliary cirrhosis, diabetes mellitus. Most of these diseases are associated with T-lymphocyte defects.

*Vitamin C,*
*Zinc, B₆, and*
*Linoleic Acid*
*Work Together*

According to Horrobin, prostaglandin (PG) EI plays a major role in regulating thymus development and in the function of T-lymphocytes. Most important, the production of PG EI is highly dependent on various nutritional factors, including vitamin C, zinc, pyridoxine, and the fatty acids gamma-linolenic acid and linoleic acid. The author contends that an inadequate intake of any one of these nutrients will "lead to inadequate PG EI formation and defective T-lymphocyte function." Further, "Megadoses of any one are likely to be only minimally effective in the absence of adequate intakes of the others. By careful attention to diet, it should be possible to activate T-lymphocyte function." These nutrients are commonly available in fresh fruits, vegetables, whole grains, and fresh meat. Vegetable oils such as safflower, soy, corn, and peanut supply the necessary fatty acids. Note that these foods are commonly available in many traditional menus, and seriously lacking in deethnicized, processed foods.

*Immune*
*System*
*Bolstered by*
*Common*
*Nutrients*

The efficiency of the immune system is intimately interconnected with the production of PG EI and its stimulating effect on the production of T-lymphocytes. This possibility is strongly suggested by related evidence. For example, glucocorticoids tend to inhibit PG EI formation and cause "dramatic thymus atrophy." Also, lithium, which is used for treating manic-depressive disorders, inhibits the formation of PG EI when found in concentrations necessary for treating this disorder. Further, ascorbic acid is involved intimately in the production of a "thymic humoral factor." It is important to remember that too high a dosage of various drugs that overproduce PG EI can work to reduce the efficiency of the immune system and create adverse effects. Horrobin states, "Clearly much work remains to be done in sorting out precisely the effects of PG EI (and of other PGs) on the individual components of the immune system. Such biphasic effects may help to explain why penicillamine and levamisole have proved such extraordinarily difficult drugs to manage, particularly in relation to dosage." But apparently we need not worry about overdosing on these nutritional factors which stimulate the production of lymphocytes. Drugs may override control mechanisms, but it is unlikely that nutrients do likewise; and so on a preventive basis it is important that we receive adequate quantities of essential fatty acids, vitamin B₆, zinc, and vitamin C—nutrients whose intake is marginal or deficient in most Western diets. Specific amounts of these nutrients are described in detail in the chapter "Computing Your Own Nutritional Needs." At this time we must look at other leads linking diet, nutrition, and cancer.

# Herbal Remedies Against Cancer

It is unknown at this time whether plants reputed for antineoplastic properties work because of the chlorophyll they contain or by other mechanisms. The Hoxie Clinic in Texas has long touted red clover as a principal ingredient in their anticancer infusion. Other plants of high regard in American folklore for anticancer activity include chaparral. Of course there are other plants in many parts of the world that have been used against cancer. It would be ludicrous for me to suggest that only drugs of plant origin will ultimately cure the multiplicity of diseases known as cancer; but there are products presently available derived from plants which hold great promise in controlling one of these diseases—leukemia. In fact, vincristine, obtained from the periwinkle, is one of the most important drugs used in treating acute childhood leukemia, and is also the therapy of choice in some other kinds of malignant disease.

*Standard Leukemia Remedy Derived from Tropical Periwinkle*

Of the several thousand plant species known to have been used since ancient Egyptian times, over 100,000 plant materials were screened for anticancer activity at the National Cancer Institute. While this fascinating antitumor program has yielded some remarkable drugs of potential clinical value, the subject is worthy of another book and will only be mentioned in passing.

A recent literature search pointed out that there are more than eleven hundred species of plants known to have antitumor properties. Scientific investigation of a few of these plants led to some fifty chemical compounds that have gone or will soon go into clinical trial against human neoplastic diseases. Of the thousands of plants mentioned in the folklore of various countries as having been used for treating cancer, a high percentage have been shown to be active tumor inhibitors. These folkloric anticancer remedies, such as *Aristolochia indica, Asclepias curassavica, Podophyllum peltatum, Sanguinaria canadensis, Solanum dulcamara, Acnistus arborescens,* and *Senecio triangularis,* have all been found to contain cytotoxic and/or antitumor principles. Thus folklore is a highly predictive tool for selecting potential anticancer drugs. Other plants from folklore used for treating some of the more than two hundred different types of cancer include henna, horehound, juniper berries, mezereon, and Solomon's seal. These plants have been treated in greater detail in an earlier work,* and the reader is referred to this book for a more complete discussion.

*Many Plants Demonstrate Anticancer Activity*

The more than 500,000 higher plant species on the planet Earth certainly may hold a cure for some forms of this disease, and mankind has turned to the earth in his search from earliest times. The Ebers Papyrus, which dates from about 1550 B.C., contains the earliest known record of the use of plants for treating cancerlike diseases. More than forty different plants are recommended in this early Egyptian work for treating tumors, warts, and other malignant growths. Plants recommended include barley, garlic, flax, coriander, figs, onions, absinth, papyrus, dates, and grapes. While some of these recommendations were no doubt fanciful, it is interesting that this ancient work also recommended juniper berries. Juniper produces a substance that is selectively toxic to cancer cells. Also this ancient manuscript recommended yeast, a rich source of folic acid. This suggestion led to the use of folic acid antagonists in cancer therapy.

One of the most potent tumor inhibitors to be derived from the world of plants is vincristine, isolated from the Madagascan periwinkle, *Catharanthus roseus (Vinca rosea)*. This plant, and the drugs derived from it, is one of the most interesting stories about the role of chance in the development of effective chemotherapeutic agents.

The story was first told by Noble, et al., in 1958. While extracts of the periwinkle had been used as early as 1653 for treating gingivitis and diabetes, it was more than three hundred years later that the antitumor properties of these extracts were noted. As Dr. Noble tells it:

The chain of events . . . originated in our laboratory in 1949 because we had been working with, and were somewhat intrigued by, various plant extracts to which historical hearsay had ascribed empirical uses by primitive peoples. The disease of cancer was certainly far from our thoughts when we learned of a tea made from the leaves of a West Indian shrub that was supposedly useful in the control of diabetes mellitus. C. D. Johnston of Black River, Jamaica, Federated West Indies, had been curious about the reputed benefits of a tea made from the leaves of the white flowered periwinkle, *Vinca rosea;* he forwarded a supply of the material to us.

Although plant extracts given orally to experimental animals did not demonstrate strong hypoglycemic activity, sharp-eyed

* *Weiner's Herbal* (New York: Stein & Day, 1980).

researchers recognized that those animals who received extracts of the periwinkle benefited by "some barrier to infection." Some rats developed endogenous infections that elevated the white blood count and profoundly depressed bone marrow. A water extract of 2 grams of the dried leaves of periwinkle significantly reduced the white blood count and brought about a virtual disappearance of neutrophil leukocytes. Further studies demonstrated that a component of the periwinkle extract was responsible for this activity. This component was eventually isolated and termed vinblastine. Workers in another laboratory soon found that periwinkle extracts had definite activity against leukemia. This led to the isolation of another alkaloid, vincristine. While both alkaloids are similar in their activity against experimental animal tumors, they differ markedly in their reactions in man and in their toxic effects. Vincristine induces a 90 percent response rate when administered in conjunction with corticosteroids in treating acute lymphocytic leukemia. It is also used for treating Hodgkin's disease and Wilms's tumor. Vincristine does not depress bone marrow function; however, it does cause some neurotoxicity, constipation, and a loss of deep tendon reflexes. And so, while not without their side effects, two of our most potent anticancer drugs—available to physicians for many years—were derived from herbal remedies well known to folklore.

# Nutrition and Cancer Around the World*

In November of 1975 a symposium sponsored by the American Cancer Society and the National Cancer Institute addressed itself to the question of nutrition in the causation of cancer. Represented were researchers from around the world, who approached the many types of cancer from an epidemiological standpoint. Different groups discussed various aspects of the disease, such as alcoholism and its relationship to cancer in terms of nutritional imbalance, and cancer of the upper alimentary tract as related to certain foods in different parts of the world. The question of hormone-dependent cancers as related to dietary factors was treated, as were dietary factors in cancer of the large bowel, cancers of the pancreas and stomach, and miscellaneous dietary factors.

Having read all of the published papers from this confer-

---

* See *Cancer Research*, Volume 35(11): 3231–3550 (1975). This volume contains all papers I refer to in this section.

ence, certain conclusions could be drawn or inferred which may be useful to those interested in lessening the likelihood of developing any form of this dread disease. In what follows much speculation is apparent; the individual bias is often elevated to the status of a hypothesis with somewhat makeshift experimental evidence. Nevertheless we must accept the sense of things, the feelings of the conference's participants for their subject. If not "truth," then a summary of the articles that appeared following this conference provides a set of coordinates through which a line may be drawn. It is up to the reader to draw an arrowhead.

*Science and Art Interrelated*

What does this foggy situation indicate—a lack of ability on the part of the cited workers, or the tremendous complexity of the subject matter? I think neither. For me, science is at its most lucid an elegant expression of an idea. True, there is a method to the scientific exposition, but in the final analysis it is just man's ideas we are dealing with. How does the scientist differ from the artist in his expression of ideas? Both seek to communicate a special idea or insight, yet their methods of statement obviously differ. While the scientist offers proof in the form of experimental or statistical evidence, the artist attempts this "proof" by sheer control of his medium. The painting, sculpture, musical score, manuscript, is offered as proof. By its elegance of execution it communicates the special idea. Yet the question of adequate proof troubles the scientist. Albeit elegant, many scientific proofs fail to convince on intimate analysis. In light of the limitations inherent in the nature of science, which is itself a theory, the following summary represents what is to me a series of interesting ideas about nutritional factors in cancer.

*Some Cancers Caused by Known Factors*

It may be best to begin by paraphrasing an early worker in the field of environmentally induced cancers, Dr. Heuper. This insightful researcher long ago stated that cancer is not a mysterious disease of unknown origin; rather, he reasoned, it is a disease caused by many known compounds. Dr. Heuper then went on to cite numerous occupational relationships to various forms of this disease. For example, rubber workers, polyvinyl chloride workers, creosote workers, and those working in the asbestos industries unfortunately have much higher incidences of various cancers than the population at large. But Dr. Heuper was not the first to tie in environment and disease. From many early sources, and we might add, in most primitive cultures, we learn that mankind has long associated disease states with living habits, including food. Thus many religions have strict dietary laws, and as we shall soon see with the Seventh-Day Adventists, who follow many reasonable dietary laws, there may be evidence to support the contention that adherence to diet-related religious laws is rewarded with a lessened incidence of cancer.

Much scientific work in the area of diet and cancer was undertaken in the post–World War II period, when a multitude of new and unproven chemicals began to appear in the food supply. Beginning with intuitive ideas, several workers attempted to show cause-and-effect relationships between some of these food chemicals and various cancers. (At this time only a few studies, dating back only ten or so years, will be cited.) Thus in 1964 the possibility that charcoal broiling created some carcinogen was reported in *Science* magazine. The subject was again reviewed in a more recent issue of *Science,* where it was stated that charcoal broiling often produces considerable benzo-a pyrine content in broiled meat. Publication of the fact that such carcinogenic polynuclear hydrocarbons are produced in the cooking of food was a landmark in the field.

*Charcoal Broiling Produces Carcinogens on Food*

To put this matter in perspective, polycyclic hydrocarbons also occur naturally in many foods and as a result of processing. Tea, for example, has been found to contain about 0.04 microgram ($\mu$g) of carcinogens (per average daily intake), comparable to that from coffee (0.05 $\mu$g) and bread (0.05 $\mu$g), but less than the amount found in green vegetables (0.15–4.0 $\mu$g) and *much less* than the amount found in barbecued meat (1000 $\mu$g!) (Stagg and Millin, 1975).

"Ethnic" dietetics can be seen to play a significant role in determining how much of this carcinogen people ingest. Teas from Japan contain levels of 3,4-benzpyrene similar to Assam tea, while black tea has considerably *lower* amounts of DDT than Japanese green tea. People who *broil* meat and fish generally ingest higher quantities of carcinogens than those who bake or boil their foods—the cooking method often determined by ethnic or cultural preferences.

*Baked and Boiled Foods Safer*

Another cooking relationship to cancer was published in 1969 by O'Gara and workers, who concluded that "the continual heating of hydrogenated fat may cause cancer-inciting substances to be formed." This implied a relationship between much-used cooking oil and cancer. Therefore fried foods, especially those served in fast-food restaurants where oil is repeatedly reused, are to be avoided!

Two years earlier, in 1967, Epstein and coworkers had indicated that the herbicide maleic hydrazide, which is used to inhibit sprouting on many root crops, caused cancer in test animals. Incidentally, this maleic hydrazide is sprayed on potatoes and appears in our finished foods.

In the past few years the literature on nutritional relationships to cancer has grown enormously. Many recent studies and publications deal with cancer of the large bowel, or colon. This is so because in Great Britain and the United States cancer of the large bowel is second only to lung cancer as a cause of death; but mortality from it differs in different parts of the world. Furthermore, internationally there is a correlation between the mortality rates for colon cancer and coronary heart disease. A current theory is that dietary fat is suspected as a common etiological factor, both in coronary heart disease and bowel cancer, perhaps operating in colon cancer through the transformation of bile salts into carcinogens by certain intestinal bacteria.

## Bowel Gas and Carcinogenesis

*Cultural Factors Influence Amount of Bowel Gas Retained*

My hypothesis is that those of us who tend to suppress the impulse to "pass gas" run a greater risk of contracting cancer of the large bowel and rectum than those of us who release at will. This tends to be supported by statistics from various countries where cultural attitudes affect individual action or suppression in this matter. Japanese, for example, think nothing of passing gas at a good dinner, something a "proper" North American, Dane, or Britisher would never dare do. The incidence of large bowel and rectal cancer is greatest in the "uptight" countries and lowest in nations where there seems to be less of a "hang-up" about one's own bodily functions (Africa, India, Singapore, Chile, and Japan; see table, "Regional Variations in Cancer Incidence").

This variation in incidence of bowel cancer has been explained as having to do with the amount of meat people eat (the more meat the greater the risk of bowel cancer), and also related to the relative amount of fibrous foods eaten (the more fiber, the lower the incidence of bowel cancer). I suspect that carcinogenesis in the large bowel is also related to the amount of gas one holds in this organ. Methane, or "swamp gas," is a major component of bowel gas. When it reacts with chlorine in the large bowel (a product of water treatment), hydrochloric acid and a free radical are formed, as shown in the following formula:

$$CH_4 \quad + Cl \quad \longrightarrow HCl \qquad + \text{free radical}$$
(methane)   (chlorine)   (hydrochloric
                       acid)

This free radical then reacts with another molecule, producing *another* free radical. This self-propagating chain reaction continues until all materials are consumed or until two free radicals meet and join, producing, perhaps, carcinogenic substances that initiate the process of bowel cancer. Thus, in addition to implicating bowel gas in this process, I suspect that the chlorination of water also contributes to this disease process, as described above. Of course, potent carcinogens such as methyl chloride, chloroform, and carbon tetrachloride are also produced when methane is chlorinated, as any first-year chemistry student learns. To protect yourself from speeding this process, I can only suggest that you excuse yourself from the dinner table, leave the room, not hesitating for a minute out of polite considerations, a frequent enemy of the natural man within.

Having reviewed the papers at the Nutrition in the Causation of Cancer conference, the following summaries are worth mentioning.

1. Alcohol may be a very important cofactor in the origin of head and neck cancers in the United States and Western Europe. It seems that excessive alcohol ingestion, coupled with nutritional deficiency or smoking, may be carcinogenic. Further, alcohol in excessive amounts may suppress immune systems. A number of vitamin and mineral deficiencies are also associated with excessive alcohol ingestion. It seems that alcohol either removes the following minerals and vitamins, or inhibits their development within the body: thiamine, folic acid, magnesium, iron, pyridoxine, pantothenic acid, riboflavin, zinc, and copper.

It is thought that alcohol may convert a procarcinogen into a carcinogen, or that the distilling process itself may produce potential carcinogens, as for example, fusel oil, which is a by-product of distillation. Further, the process of aging whiskey in charcoal-lined barrels containing various polycyclic hydrocarbons, for which alcohol is an excellent solvent, might produce carcinogens in these beverages. *Fusel Oil in Whiskey Dangerous*

2. It is pretty well established that many food additives have strong potential as carcinogens. In an excellent review by Dr. Shubik entitled "The Potential Carcinogenicity of Food Addi- *Food Additives Implicated*

## Regional Variations in Cancer Incidence

| Site | High Incidence | Medium Incidence | Low Incidence |
|---|---|---|---|
| Skin (males) | Southern Europe, USA, Canada, Australia, Colombia, Puerto Rico | Northern and Central Europe, United Kingdom | Africa, Japan, Singapore (Chinese) |
| Mouth excluding lip (males) | Ceylon, India | France | Most countries |
| Lung (males) | United Kingdom, Germany, Finland, USA | Latin America, Japan, Denmark, Iceland, Norway, Canada | Africa, India |
| Esophagus (males) | Japan, China, Southern Africa, Jamaica, Iran, Southern USSR, Caribbean area | France, Switzerland, Singapore, India, Chile | North America, Most European countries, Israel |
| Stomach | Japan, Chile, Iceland, Colombia, Finland, Newfoundland, USSR | Most European countries, Canada, Caribbean area | Africa, USA, India |
| Large bowel and rectum | North America, Denmark, United Kingdom | Israel, Finland, Iceland, Argentina | Africa, India, Singapore, Chile, Japan |
| Nasopharynx (males) | Singapore (Chinese), Southern China | Malaya, Thailand, Indonesia, Kenya | Europe, Africa (most areas), India |
| Liver (males) | Mozambique, Southern Africa | Japan, Singapore (Chinese), Nigeria, Uganda | North America, Europe, Jamaica, South America, India |
| Body of uterus (females) | Europe, North America, Israel | Jamaica, Puerto Rico, Chile, Japan | Southern Africa, Nigeria |
| Cervix (females) | Colombia, Puerto Rico, Southern Africa, Jamaica, USA (nonwhite) | West and East, Africa, Japan, Singapore (Chinese), India, Europe | United Kingdom, Israel (very rare), USA (white), New Zealand |
| Breast (females) | North America, Europe | Colombia, Jamaica, Chile, India, Yugoslavia | Japan, Africa, Singapore (Chinese) |

FROM Higginson, 1968.

tives and Contaminants," the following key points are made: (a) While tests for carcinogenicity are often in conflict on the same substances, this does not mean that a green light should be given every compound. In fact, overt carcinogenicity of a compound is easily handled. The compound is banned for use in food. "It is when borderline results occur repeatedly that serious problems arise." As an example, the cyclamates are discussed, and here the author believes "that an error was made originally when cyclamate was allowed on the market in the United States without having been tested properly." (b) Shubik also points out that vitamin C inhibits nitrosamines. He calls for detailed investigation of the compounds such as vitamin C which have the potential of being able to neutralize carcinogenic food additives or inhibit their formation. We might add that, as already noted, Linus Pauling first suggested an anticancer role for this vitamin in 1974, in his paper, "Ascorbic Acid and the Glycosominoglycans: A Contribution to the Orthomolecular Treatment of Cancer." (c) Shubik offers the interesting suggestion that more attention be paid "to cooking procedures of which smoking is one. The vast number of things that may occur in cooking constitute a Pandora's box just waiting to be opened by some fortunate young scientist who is going to make a name for himself in the future." (d) Shubik also brought out the effects of arsenic and the excessive use of iron in our diet. He states that "there are a variety of iron derivatives that have been shown to produce tumors in animals." He then cites the case where ferrous gluconate is used in California to make black olives "shiny black."

3. Some of the most interesting papers at the Nutrition and Cancer Symposium were those epidemiological studies culled from around the world. A few key points will serve to elucidate these.

Workers in the Caspian littoral of Iran found striking variations in the incidence of esophageal cancer in a three-hundred-mile area of Iran. These varied as much as thirtyfold in women and sixfold in men. It was found that the cancer rates in the Gonbad region are among the highest reported for this tumor in the entire world. The main dietary factors isolated were the fact that white bread is eaten instead of rice as a food staple; a large amount of sheep and goat's milk or yogurt is used; there is a lack of fruits or vegetables eaten, with a corresponding low intake of vitamin A, vitamin C, and riboflavin. The workers emphasized that bread may be a key factor here. "Some households had nothing but bread, sugar, and tea for

*Iranian Diet No Longer Balanced*

the entire five days of the dietary study. Hot tea cannot be responsible as the main factor." They concluded that "a restricted diet renders the population highly susceptible."

*Aflatoxins in Thai and African Diets*

Liver cancer in Thailand and Africa was evaluated by Dr. Wogan and coworkers. In Africa liver cancer in Swaziland and Uganda is related to aflatoxins in beans, maize, and sorghum. Aflatoxins are defined by the National Academy of Sciences as follows:

The word is used in a generic sense to designate some ten or more brightly fluorescing furanocoumarin compounds of which aflatoxin B is a prototype. They are hepatotoxic—carcinogenic metabolites of Aspergillus flavus and of closely related fungi that grow on many different foodstuffs when sufficient moisture is present.

Going back to studies on liver cancer in Thailand and Africa, it was found that in Thailand "aflatoxin concentration in what superficially seemed to be wholesome foods or foodstuffs destined for human consumption were as high as 772 parts per billion (ppb) in dried fish; 996 ppb in dried chili peppers; 2.7 parts per million (ppm) in corn, and more than 2 ppm in peanuts." While these values appear to be quantitatively small, these compounds are extremely potent. We must ask if the peanuts, corn, and dried vegetables grown and stored in America are free of aflatoxins.

Based upon these and other studies, such as those in Mozambique, which has the highest known incidence of liver cancer in the world, that is, 25.4 deaths per 100,000 per year, the authors conclude that "there is a significant correlation between the levels of aflatoxin consumption and liver cancer incidence." While this is not based on unequivocal proof, the data are nevertheless significant. It should be remembered that it is unlikely that aflatoxin B is carcinogenic per se. This potent toxin must be metabolically activated to be carcinogenic and to be reactive *in vivo*.

*Adventists Rewarded for Moderation and Abstinence*

4. Perhaps one of the most interesting studies reported at the conference was that of Dr. Phillips and coworkers on the "Role of Lifestyle and Dietary Habits in Risk of Cancer Among Seventh-Day Adventists." It is well known that Seventh-Day Adventists abstain from smoking and drinking; about 50 percent follow a lacto-ovo vegetarian diet; and most avoid the use of coffee, tea, hot condiments, and spices. With regard to cancer rates, the mortality rates are 50 to 70 percent of general population rates for most cancer sites unrelated to drinking and smoking. But this "may be due to selective factors," for example,

socioeconomic status and education, which could be related to dietary habits as well.

This "selective factor" hypothesis was further examined by comparing mortality rates of physicians, one group Adventists and the other non-Adventists, who were graduates of University of Southern California Medical School. It was found that death rates in physicians of both groups are much *lower* than the general population rates, but surprisingly, mortality rates in both groups of physicians, Adventists and non-Adventists, are essentially the same for all causes and all cancers. With these restrictions, Dr. Phillips offers that the low fat and cholesterol and high fiber of the Adventist diet may relate to lower cancer risks; second, that lack of coffee consumption by most Adventists might account for reduced bladder cancer risk; third, that using fewer refined and processed foods than the general public, lower exposure to carcinogenic food additives or contaminants results. Fourth, their ability to handle nitrosamines, aflatoxin, polycyclic hydrocarbons, might be greater due to relatively high intake of vitamin C and vitamin A, both of which are potentially protective against certain chemical carcinogens. Fifth, several fruits and vegetables abundantly used by Adventists contain flavones and other compounds that are potent inducers of the enzyme system involved in detoxifying absorbed carcinogens. Sixth, very low intake of animal protein by the Adventists could enable the immunological system to recognize and destroy small early clones of tumor cells:

*Low Animal Protein, Low Fat, High Fiber, Fresh Foods Advised*

This possibility is particularly attractive because of the rather general decrease in cancer mortality from almost all cancer sites in Adventists, which is more suggestive of a stronger defense system against cancer than lack of exposure to a few of the known multiple environmental carcinogens.

It is no longer necessary to look upon cancer as an act of God, nor even as essentially a legacy from our ancestors. The evidence incriminating the sophisticated environment as the essential and most easily corrected cause has become more and more compelling.

—SHENNAN AND BISHOP, 1974

## Diets Around the World

In looking at cancer and diet in thirty-two countries, the above workers drew some clear conclusions: (1) carcinomas of the upper alimentary tract, larynx, uterine body, thyroid, and liver are unrelated to food factors; (2) carcinoma of the nose and nasal sinuses is associated with deficiency of food of all the main calorie-rich types; and, most interestingly, (3) "In the majority of cases the main emphasis is on fats. In others it is on sugar and total calories. In a few instances protein intake is among the factors highly related. All these may be considered together as a 'dietary' group though fat and oil consumption has the highest and most constant association."

*Fats Accelerate Tumor Growth*    The work of Shennan and Bishop is based upon an earlier literature review done by Poulson (1949), who reviewed the literature on the relationship between the growth of tumors and dietary manipulation in rats. He found that "it is strikingly clear that if the administration of calories is reduced the incidence of spontaneous tumors as well as of tumors accelerated by hydrocarbons decreases and the age of occurrence increases." Also:

> A diet rich in fat exerts an accelerating action on the development of spontaneous as well as carcinogenically accelerated tumors. The action besides the purely caloric action may in a way be attributed to the local action of fat on the resorption of the carcinogen, but there is apparently also a specific action of the genuine fats as such which seems to follow the fatty acid radicals.

Poulson stated that as early as 1911 it was already known that "all substances known to be capable of giving rise to atypical epithelial growth had one common property, namely that they were soluble in fatty substances and fat solvents."

*Environmental Factors More Important Than Ethnic*    In a study, "Role of Ethnic Background in Cancer Development," by Baruch Modan (1974), relative rates of various malignant disorders among different ethnic groups in Israel were studied. Compared were European-born with Asian- and African-born groups. A striking parallel to patterns of cancer seen in white and black groups in the United States was noticed. The authors conclude:

> Since the Israel and American ethnic subgroups do not have a common genetic background, it would seem that the similarities observed are associated with interethnic differences in socioeconomic status. This corroborates previous observations on the role of environmental factors in carcinogenesis.

Hence Modan concludes that ethnic factors are not as significant as environmental factors in the development of various cancers. According to this study the socioeconomic factor is the most important because factors underlying this influence vary from cancer site to cancer site, and include fertility patterns, occupation, and diet. Differences *do* occur in the risk of cancer in different sites among different groups in Israel. For example, esophageal cancer rates are very low in North African–born people, while this tumor is particularly frequent among Yemenites and Iranians in that country. Cancer of the larynx seems to occur more frequently amongst immigrants from Bulgaria, Greece, and Turkey, and the authors conclude that "the general and probably oversimplified socioeconomic gradient hypothesis does not apply to all cancer categories." He goes on to suggest that for some cancer sites genetically determined characteristics may play a role, suggesting further that a G6PD deficiency (see Chapter 3) or other biochemical components are involved. Certainly diet is not to be ruled out, because smoking and drinking of tannin-rich hot teas must certainly play a role in various cancers and various sites.

Modan attempts to rule out a common genetic background for comparable subgroups in Israel and the USA, but omits the possibility that the American black population and the black people in Israel might possibly have emigrated or originated from a similar genetic pool. He states that the American black population "originated from Central Africa," while the black and Oriental population in Israel "immigrated from North Africa and the Middle East." These statements are true unto themselves, as are the geographies of origin; however, going into the far distant past, prior to historical records, it is possible that the black population of America and a segment of the non-European population in Israel may have common genetic origins, which would tend to support the genetic theory. There is some chance that the Falashas, or black Jews of Ethiopia, and some American blacks share similar origins.

*Origin of Gene Pools Examined*

# Beyond Laetrile

While the preceding summary of papers at the Nutrition and Cancer conference has largely been an exploration of nutritional *causes* of cancer in conjunction with other factors, it may be interesting to raise a few questions regarding the nutritional *defenses* against this disease state.

According to the proponents of laetrile, for example, certain specific foods may be protective against cancer. Laetrile is essentially amygdalin, a glycoside or sugar found in many foods, which breaks down into hydrocyanic acid or cyanide (HCN)

*Laetrile Hypothesis Examined*

inside the cell. The supporters of laetrile therapy argue that HCN is harmless to healthy cells but toxic to cancer cells, which are rapidly developing and hypersensitive to this potent chemical. Theoretically at least the argument is interesting. For those interested in possibly insulating themselves against this dread disease, the following is a list of foods which contain amygdalin: these include all members of the rose family, almond, apple, apricot, cherry, peach, pear, plum, and quince. Other foods which yield high HCN include buckwheat, millet, flaxseed, elderberry jelly, plum jam, lima beans, bean sprouts, sorghum, molasses, cashew nuts, and the liqueur kirsch, which is made from cherries. It is interesting how few of these foods are eaten in any quantity in our contemporary diets, but that they once did comprise a substantial portion of man's daily bread. If there is some way to evaluate the incidence of cancer in populations that consume large quantities of some of these foods, we could possibly decide if the laetrilists have something in their interesting proposal.

*Are Apricots Protective?*    The study that we would propose might take place among the Hunza people of the Himalayas, who are reputedly quite healthy and long lived. They subsist to a great extent on dried apricots during the long winter months. The pits of apricots, which are seen as unfit for human consumption elsewhere due to the high HCN levels, are consumed as nuts to supplement the sparse diet. Questions to answer would be: (1) What is the relative incidence of cancer among the Hunzas? (2) How much HCN is ingested annually by the Hunza population? (3) Are the apricot pits prepared prior to consumption? Certainly too many variables exist even to suggest a relationship, but these fragments of the puzzle would be worth elucidating. Perhaps working among the Hunzas would stimulate further thought. It is certainly reasonable to study the healthiest, most disease-free people, rather than focusing on those who are diseased.

Other groups worth investigating are those who eat cassava, rich also in cyanogenetic glycosides—groups such as those in Nigeria and regions of South America where types of cassava rich in HCN are to be found. Such studies must be undertaken *before* any inordinate quantities of cyanide-yielding foods are taken on a cancer preventive hypothesis.

# Book Four

# NOON CLARITY

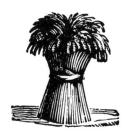

# 12 AT THE NUTRITIONIST'S

The first thing you must consider when shopping for a nutritionist who can act positively to maintain and restore optimal health is the kind of education and training he or she has had. This, like all "new age" medical and paramedical fields, is fast becoming flooded with the flotsam and jetsam of would-be experts, including physicians with little formal training in a sepecialty as demanding as surgery, pathology, gastroenterology, and others.

Nutrition as a specialty is today where psychiatry was when Freud took his medical degree, one hundred years ago, in 1881. At this time, while there are no state or federal requirements for a field in transition, there are definite screening tools *you* can employ to separate the best practitioners from the near imposters.

## The Ideal Nutritionist

Many "nutritionists" claim miracles from specialized diets that they claim to have discovered. Unfortunately almost all of these alleged benefits are anecdotal. When suffering from some illness or disability, many of us seek magic, hoping that the "expert" advocating the cure is honest and knowledgeable, and not merely an exploiter.

### Food Combinations

We see many suggestions for maximizing health and longevity, perhaps the most bizarre being various concepts regarding the restriction of intake of protein foods with carbohydrates, in the same meal. There is no reason to believe we must segregate proteins from carbohydrates in the same meal.

*New Food*
*Prohibitions*
*Questioned*

If various individuals propose this restrictive combination and, further, offer literally dozens of combinations that they have "discovered" to be especially health-inducing, then perhaps we might all seek their counsel, for who knows, a new nutritional messiah may be in our midst. After all, it took only fifteen thousand years of experiments for the Meso-Americans eventually to find the bean-corn diet; perhaps our new messiah has been able to speed the process somewhat, giving us new and wondrous food combinations after only a few years of thought! If this be the case, we must address ourselves to this long-awaited messiah at once.

I do not mean to imply by this that there are not many people who are sincere in their belief that they have found certain magical combinations in foods and wish to give these to the world. But very frequently the leaders are as much in error as those who subscribe to and practice their theories. Furthermore, the mere fact that an individual may show improvement on a dietary regimen is far from scientific proof that the dietary regimen itself had a significant effect upon the disease process.

*Placebo, a*
*Strong Factor*

Being involved in a therapeutic relationship will result in a significant number of people showing improvement, irrespective of the disease process itself. This has been confirmed repeatedly, and the percentage of improvement varies with both the nature of the illness and the personalities of the therapist and the patient, ranging from as low as a 20 percent response to as high as a 70 to 80 percent response. This effect has been referred to as the placebo effect, or in psychological jargon, the Hawthorne effect. The question has often been raised, "So what if the response is merely that of a placebo effect? The very fact that the individual has improved in this therapeutic situation should be sufficient evidence of the efficacy of the procedure." But from the point of view of world medicine this is not adequate. We are interested in knowing the mechanisms involved, and if the mechanisms are really due to the combination of foods or the nutrients in these foods. Then we can be relatively certain of the basic biological causes of the therapeutic action and ultimately have a better understanding of the disease. The difficulty with the placebo effect is that it is usually temporary and may well mask more serious underlying conditions, and the patient, although apparently responding, actually is deteriorating and may reach a point of no return.

We are constantly being bombarded with an increasing flow of books, as well as media exposure of personalities who make extravagant claims, advocating miraculous but simplistic cures of some of the most difficult nutritional problems of our society. How are we to decide whom we can trust and from whom we can obtain advice that is honest, current, and based upon rational principles?

While the so-called "ideal nutritionist," like the "ideal diet," does not exist, we can at least describe the characteristics of an individual whom we can trust to give us the best possible answers based on the best knowledge available at the present time. Nutrition, like all scientific fields, is a very rapidly changing one, and the honest nutritionist, first of all, would be the first to admit where a serious lack of knowledge lies and where he is making educated guesses, and second, to call attention to changes in the area of nutritional knowledge as these areas undergo change. *True Nutritionist Admits Limitations*

One of the first things we want to know regarding a professional is his or her prior training. In our society the subject of health and disease has become entrusted to people educated within the medical establishment. Unfortunately, in the case of nutrition the physician is not the proper individual to consult. The reason for this is that the field of nutrition, particularly over the last twenty-five to thirty-five years, has been very seriously neglected in medical schools. Only recently, with the recognition that about 50 percent of patients who enter hospitals have malnutrition as one of their problems, has there been a tremendous resurgence of interest in the problem of malnutrition, particularly in the major training hospitals of this country. But the shortage of trained nutritionists has been so acute that it will be many years before adequate training for physicians and others within our classical medical institutions will be able to provide us with enough professionals to give nutritional advice to individuals. For the time being, seriously malnourished patients are the only ones receiving the attention of the medical nutritionist. *Question Your Health Consultant*

## A Dietitian Is Not a Nutritionist

If we cannot look to a physician, to whom can we look? Over the years there has been a relatively large group of people whose training in nutrition has been relatively minimal. Usually known as dietitians, their requirements are four years of college, specializing in areas of nutrition, generally followed by a period of internship which usually consists of some type of service in a hospital or other health facility. These dietitians have generally not been trained in rigorous scientific techniques, and their clinical experience has been relatively limited. They have been taught primarily to help interpret nutritional information, which has already been predigested, to patients, usually on order or prescription of a physician. But until recently dietitians have taken little initiative in becoming involved in nutritional research themselves.

*Dietitians Not Trained as Nutritionists*

Dietitians probably constitute the largest numbers among the so-called therapeutic nutritionists. The advice that you are likely to receive from such individuals will usually be relatively simple, standardized medical-establishment advice, with little consideration of the tremendous impact that today's food system has had upon our food supply, and frequently with misunderstanding about the application to individuals of standards such as the RDAs, which were established for adequate nutrition of groups. A well-trained nutritionist, on the other hand, deals not only with mere nutrients, but with the whole person, including cultural beliefs about diet and health.

A third group consists of generally much better trained professionals, who usually work in public-health agencies and who often work in programs with individuals. They have usually received their dietetics training and then have gone to a school of public health where they have received a master's degree in public health. They have been trained to look at the broad problems of nutritionally implicated diseases such as obesity, diabetes, heart disease, etc. These individuals also, unfortunately, are not generally trained in depth, but they are usually at least better informed, particularly those who are trained in one of the ten schools of public health in the United States.

*Professors Not Clinicians*

Next are nutritionists who have been well trained, usually within a department of nutritional science, but who very frequently received their bachelor's degree not in nutrition but in a hard biological science, transferring to nutrition, obtaining their master's and/or doctoral degree, and then spending time in research and ultimately in teaching, and sometimes moving on to clinical work in the area of nutrition. Not all of these individuals are free of suspicion, but in general one can say that these professionals have a broader view of nutrition. Unfortunately, although they would undoubtedly deny this, many university-affiliated nutritionists receive considerable support from the food industry.* While they may attempt to do their

* The recent disclosure that some members of the Food and Nutrition Board of the National Academy of Sciences receive up to 10 percent of their income from industry is a case in point. Here, some "objective" scientists are on the payroll of the egg, dairy, sugar, and beef "advisory boards."

research in a highly scientific and "objective" manner, it is well documented that there is no scientific experiment that does not contain built-in bias. When the bias comes as a result of support from funds generated by a group like the food industry, which might have ulterior motives in supporting such research, individuals who receive such support, and the conclusions of experiments supported by industry, must of necessity remain suspect in the mind of the public.

Having gone down our list, we find that our quest for the helpful empathetic nutritionist is not a simple one; but there are individuals to whom we can at least turn for information. However, whenever we do so we must also understand that even the advice given to us by the most highly trained and highly respected professional must be understandable to us and acceptable to us, both at an intellectual level and at a gut level, before we can accept the information which we have received.

# At the Nutritionist's

After finding your nutritionist, possibly to gauge your present state of nutritional knowledge, to evaluate your diet, or to have specific ailments treated, you can expect an initial evaluation of approximately one hour. What goes into and what leaves your digestive system is the province of the nutritionist. A complete evaluation of your nutritional status may begin with data forms such as the following (employed in my clinical practice).

## Overview to Services You Can Expect

### Why You May Need the Services of a Nutritionist

Food and drinks, or the absence of such, are the number one factors in our personal health care. What we choose to eat, when we choose to eat (or not eat), and how we eat can alter our perceptions, affect our mood, increase or decrease our capacity to function, and greatly affect the outcome of many disease states.

By analyzing your food patterns we can construct a food and drink pattern that suits your needs. We do not believe in "food fascism" and will not give you a meal-to-meal diet unless you specifically request it. We believe in working with your established food likes and dislikes and modifying the relative proportions, to adjust the relative amounts

*Nutrition Is*
*Multifactorial*

of protein, fat, carbohydrate, and micronutrients you receive. To do this we ask you to fill out a highly detailed, computerized dietary analysis. It will come back telling us how much of your diet is composed of fats, how much of proteins, the same for carbohydrates, vitamins, minerals, and so on. Your average daily exercise and activity profile will tell us just how many calories (on the average) you expend, and, calculating this against your caloric intake, we can determine how much food you need to eliminate, and how many more minutes of each activity you need to increase to maintain or decrease your weight.

Before doing this we will want to talk about your ethnic background as it affects your food choices. We do not believe in simple, doctrinaire nutrition approaches and will not automatically tell you to stop eating pasta simply because it is made of white dough. We also must ask what emotional or cultural values this pasta has for you, before deciding to eliminate it. Further, we will want to analyze your childhood, and adolescent food likes and dislikes in creating your optimum diet. My extensive training in anthropology and work with primitive groups in the South Pacific gives me a unique opportunity to help you see what values foods may have other than their nutritional values. That is, there is more to nutrition than biochemicals, and I am trained in analyzing for these factors.

Some specific things you may want to see me for follow:

HYPOGLYCEMIA    Mood swings, aggressive/depressive episodes.

LOW ENERGY    Sharp drop in energy at 10:30 A.M. and/or 2:00 to 4:00 P.M.

ALCOHOL DEPENDENCY    Can you alter your needs through diet?

VITAMINS    Do you need them, and in what dosage? When to take them.

CHILD'S DIET    How to get them to eat the right way.

OLD AGE    What you can do to age less dramatically.

CONSTIPATION    How to control it.

MENSTRUATION    How herbs can help regulate your cycle.

MENU SUGGESTIONS

# A Problem with Computerized Dietary Analysis

While I utilize such data analysis in my practice, a limitation exists which must be explained. These forms evaluate the person's dietary intake against the standards defined by the RDAs, or Recommended Dietary Allowances. Theoretically the RDA is a good idea. Unfortunately, individuals differ. As we have seen, the RDA is valid over a broad population, but has no validity when applied to a given individual. Therefore, we must look at the RDAs as *subsistence levels* only, not *recommended* allowances. Further, when you check off the various foods you eat, bear in mind that the results of the computerized analysis are entirely dependent on the accuracy *you* bring to filling out the form.

When the form is returned, it will show how much of your daily diet consists of protein, fat, and carbohydrate, as well as how much of the known vitamins and minerals you are receiving from your foods (not including supplements). These values are generally compared with RDAs, and must be somewhat loosely interpreted, allowing for individual requirements and possible errors in completing the form.

Other data forms follow.

## Nutritional Questionnaire (for new clients)

I. *General*

Past Medical History (height, weight, physical status, etc.)

Major illnesses?

Family History (mother, father, and siblings)

Vitamins, Minerals, and Other Supplements You Take Regularly (list):
Multivitamin/Mineral: (a) brand (b) dosage
Vitamin C (dosage)
Vitamin B-Complex (dosage)
Vitamin E (dosage)
Zinc (dosage)
Others . . .

Herbal Teas You Drink Regularly? (brand name; blend of ————, ————, ————)

Allergies (list)

Foods You Crave?

Foods You Detest?

II. *Drug-Induced Nutrient Deficiencies* (after Roe, 1976.)
Are you presently taking (or within the past 3 months) any drug or home remedy for any of the health problems listed below? If yes, supply the information indicated in the table:

| Disorder | Drug Name | How Long Taken? | When Stopped? | Why Stopped? | Take Now? |
|---|---|---|---|---|---|
| Arthritis | | | | | |
| Asthma | | | | | |
| Behavior Problem | | | | | |
| Blood Clots | | | | | |
| Blood Disease | | | | | |
| Bone Disease | | | | | |
| Cholesterol (high) | | | | | |
| Colds & Sinus | | | | | |
| Colitis | | | | | |
| Constipation | | | | | |
| Convulsions | | | | | |
| Diabetes | | | | | |
| Eczema | | | | | |
| Fluid Retention | | | | | |
| Gout | | | | | |
| Headache | | | | | |
| High Blood Pressure | | | | | |
| Indigestion | | | | | |
| Insomnia | | | | | |
| Kidney Disease | | | | | |
| Liver Disease | | | | | |
| Malaria | | | | | |
| Menstrual Cramps | | | | | |
| Pain | | | | | |
| Parkinson's Disease | | | | | |
| Psoriasis | | | | | |
| Rheumatism | | | | | |
| Other (name) | | | | | |

III. *Dietary Considerations*
1. Do you see food as fuel or as a source of pleasure?
2. Do you consider yourself a fast eater, medium, or slow eater? About how many times do you *chew* each mouthful?
3. How many *full* meals do you eat daily?
4. Do you suffer from constipation? Insomnia? If so what do you take to relieve yourself?

5. How many times a week do you eat french fries?
6. How many times a week do you eat other fried foods?
7. How many times a week do you eat "fast foods"?
8. How often do you eat out? What kinds of restaurants?
9. Do you drink tea or coffee with each:
   Lunch?
   Dinner?
10. Do you add sugar or another sweetener to your hot drinks? How much?
11. Do you eat desserts? How often? Type?
12. How often do you eat ice cream?
13. How often do you eat pizza?
14. Do you eat before retiring for the night? What?
15. Do you regularly drink wine? How often?
    Domestic (brand? red, white, rosé?)
    Imported (label, type, region?)

IV. *Illness Food Choices*
Which foods or drinks did your mother or father give you for:
   (a) Sore throat?
   (b) Upset stomach?
   (c) Headache?
   (d) When you had a cold or flu?
For each of the above illnesses:
   (a) Did these foods or beverages work?
   (b) Can you speculate *why* they worked?
   (c) Which foods did not "cure" you?
   (d) Which foods made you feel worse?
   (e) How did you feel from these foods?
   (f) Can you guess why?
   (g) Do you use these foods *now* when you are sick?

V. *Food Choices for Well-Being (in childhood, and at present)*
Which foods did you eat because they were "good" for you? What did they do for you? What do they contain? Which foods did you take to *improve* some aspect of your performance? (Example: athletics, musical instrument abilities, memory, sexual prowess, and so on.) List the activity and foods you took/take to improve performance in this area.

VI. *Ethnic Food Choices*
   1. Which foods mean a great deal to you from a *family* remembrance point of view?

2. Which foods do you associate with celebrations?
3. Are these foods good for you?
4. What do you like about these foods?
5. What rituals do you perform around a meal? (Prayer, meditation, candle lighting, etc.)
6. Which foods do you avoid owing to religious beliefs? Do these have health effects?
7. Which foods do you consider "heavy" or "light?" "Hot" or "cold"? (list)
8. Do you use special utensils or dishes for different occasions? When?
9. Do you cook with gas or on an electric range? Is there a cultural reason for this?
10. How often do you serve food to other people? Do you prefer being waited on or waiting on others?

In addition to these questionnaires, your nutritionist will also likely ask you to take home a "diet diary" and carefully record your food intake for a one-week period. This will enable both of you to see at a glance patterns of significance which you may not be aware of (number of snacks, amount of wine, how much you eat after dinner, and so on). You may want to begin analyzing your own dietary patterns by filling in a daily diet survey, including all snacks. By bringing it already completed to your nutritionist you can save valuable time.

## Hair Analysis

*Hair a Health Record*

Scientists have long observed the remarkable story told by hair, but only recently has a method been developed which can isolate concentrations of elements useful in medical diagnosis. Hairs grow at a steady rate of roughly 1 centimeter per month, thus presenting a layered record of elements found *inside* the body. Hairs, like geological strata, show how substances vary in concentration over a period of time.

The most advanced method of analysis, called SAXAS (scanning automated X-ray analysis spectrometer), or X-ray fluorescence, was first developed on a large scale for the Food and Drug Administration, in conjunction with the University of Rochester. Used to detect dietary deficiencies, malabsorption syndromes, and pollutants, SAXAS is the "state of the art" in hair analysis.

*Mercury Detected in Hair*

Research engineers at California's Lawrence Berkeley Laboratory have used this technique to detect high concentrations of mercury in hair samples from Iraq. This heavy metal was absorbed by people who ate seed grain treated with a toxic fungicide. Iraqi hair samples showed a marked increase in mercury levels as comsumption of the toxic grain rose, and a gradual decline after ingestion ended.

It is significant that diet, of itself, will affect trace metal levels. In a study, "Zinc, Copper and Mercury in Oriomo Papuans' Hair" by Ohtsuka and Suzuki (1978), hair samples from the Papuans were compared between the sexes, and with those for Japanese islanders on Kuchinoshima, to the south of the Japanese mainlands. The Papuans primarily eat sago palm and meat, while the Japanese are rice- and fish-eating people. Hair zinc values of female Papuans were significantly lower than those of male Papuans and adult male and female Japanese islanders. But no difference in hair copper values was noticed. Significantly, hair organic mercury values were much *higher* in Japanese islanders than in Papuans.

*Trace Metal Levels in Hair Tell Story*

Dietary relationships explain the above findings. Female Papuans eat less meat than males, thus show lower zinc levels. The Japanese islanders eat much fish, about 111 grams daily for the male and 103 grams for the female in 1969. Very high organic mercury levels in the hair of males is directly related to the amount of fish they eat: "The low level or organic mercury in Kuchinoshima women's hair . . . [is related] to the effects of artificial hair waving in women, which *reduces* organic mercury concentrations in hair tips."

*Fish-Eaters Show High Levels of Mercury*

This important study confirms, again, the effects dietary factors play in our health, and particularly how cultural factors (i.e., Papuan males get more meat) also significantly affect nutrient levels. As we learn to interpret our own hair analysis results, we must look to the above study for some leads. For example, do you use hair dyes or shampoos which contain lead, mercury, or other elements? They may seriously affect your results and must be accounted for when you are "at the nutritionist's."

*Diet Affects Mineral Levels*

To help identify commercial products with possible high mineral contents, some hair analysis laboratories analyze many such items at no charge to their client doctors. Products must be sent to the laboratory in their original, unopened, and labeled container to ensure that the product has not been contaminated after leaving the manufacturer. A wide variety of samples have been tested, including shampoos, rinses, dyes, tints, cosmetics, ointments, and other household items. It has been found that most shampoos contain insignificant amounts of minerals with the exception of the antidandruff shampoos. These usually contain high levels of zinc and selenium. Among hair dyes and

*Limitations of Technique Described*

tints, the progressive hair darkeners which are combed in the hair daily are of major concern. These often contain very high levels of lead. (A number of facial cosmetics contain significant amounts of mercury and aluminum.)

But a few other problems with hair analysis must also be elucidated to derive the most meaningful results. We must ask if our hair truly represents our body *stores* of minerals. Or do the mineral levels present in hair simply show an *excretion* of unnecessary minerals? To correctly interpret hair analysis the nutritionist must know the entire medical history of the patient, including all supplemental minerals and drugs taken; otherwise the results may be misleading.

Also, for preventive nutritional analysis "mean values" may have no meaning for individuals with inordinate requirements for a specific mineral. For example, calcium levels for North Americans generally range between 100 to 800 parts per million (ppm) in hair, with 230 ppm the mean value. Should hair analysis show a level of 1,300 ppm, this "high" value is usually interpreted as indicative of "poor utilization by the system," on computerized printouts. The question remains, however, as to whether the individual with a high level of calcium in her hair is actually utilizing the mineral improperly, or does she have an extremely high dietary intake which is somehow required in as yet undetermined processes?

*Chest and Pubic Hair Have Limited Value*

Another problem can arise when chest and pubic hair is used for analysis. Hair from these areas grew either over a lifetime or at the time of puberty, and for a meaningful analysis of *present* mineral levels pubic or chest hair levels must be interpreted accordingly.

*Hair Analysis Has Certain Advantages*

Despite these limitations, hair analysis for trace elements has advantages over blood and urine analysis. For one, hair samples are quickly and painlessly obtained, and readily stored, transported, and analyzed. Second, mineral levels in the blood and urine are subject to daily variance, and analyzing these tissues gives us a view of minerals present only at the time of analysis. Hair, on the other hand, shows *patterns* in mineral metabolism affecting health and disease in a more consistent manner, because the hair, like fingernails or skin, contains a steady mineral supply.

TYPES OF HAIR ANALYSIS    Trace elements in human and animal hair have been studied using the following analytical methods: spectrophotometry, atomic absorption, neutron activation, spark source mass spectroscopy, and X-ray emission spectroscopy. The two most accurate methods are X-ray fluorescence (SAXAS or XRF) and inductively coupled argon plasma (ICP).

The first method, SAXAS or XRF, can detect the presence of sixteen different elements in amounts as minute as 20 millionths of a millionth of a gram (!), from hair samples as small as 2 millimeters in length. The main advantages of this method are (1) only ten strands of hair are necessary for analysis; (2) XRF is a nondestructive method; the specimens are *not* altered during analysis. Other advantages and a description of the ICP method are outlined below, as described by Mr. C. R. Alvarez, Chief Technician at Spectra Diagnostic Laboratory, San Jose, California.

## X-ray Fluorescence (XRF)

1. XRF is a nondestructive method of hair analysis.

2. This has definite advantages because the specimen is available for any number of repeat analyses. The mounted hair (only ten strands) is kept on file in the laboratory and is useful in comparative studies.

3. Normal hair growth is about 1 centimeter per month. This is of value, because we can now, to some degree, study the patient's hair as to biological time. The hair is mounted to enable us to study about 2 centimeters from the reference root. This is very helpful in monitoring either chelation therapy and/ or supplementation.

4. Many of the elements can be quantitated simultaneously, such as S, P, Ca, Ti, V, Cr, Mn, Fe, Co, Ni, Cu, Zn, As, Se, Br, Sr, Hg, Pb.

5. The coefficient of variation of Ca, Cu, Zn, S, Cl, Br, Pb, Hg, Fe, Sr are less than 15% (range 1.8–13.9). The other elements, because they are ultra trace in hair, have a higher coefficient of variation (range 18–46). These elements are near the detection limit and are only semi-quantitative; for any truly quantitative results the value of the mineral in question should be several times the detection limit.

## Inductively Coupled Argon Plasma (ICP):

1. In order to analyze hair, nails, or serum, the specimen has to be digested in acid or put into a liquid medium. This material is then atomized through a torch, reaching near 11,000° C. The combination of high temperature and a long residence

time produce complete vaporization of the sample solute and a *total breakdown* of the element under investigation into free atoms. It is then analyzed in a stable, high temperature, chemically inert zone.

2. One gram of hair is required for analysis. (Smaller amounts can be used with larger error factors.)

3. Usually about 2 inches of hair is clipped close to the scalp. This then is a representative sample of four to six months in biological time (depending on hair growth).

4. ICP instruments are excellent analyzers for trace metals regardless of manufacture. They all meet standard requirements. The problem encountered with ICP is the material that is introduced into the unit for analysis. As noted above, the sample to be analyzed has to be put into solution. Sometimes simple treatment with a solvent is sufficient, but as in the case of hair samples, more is needed. Total destruction of the organic matter is necessary. Wet oxidation is the method of choice, there being less volatilization of sought-for elements due to lower temperatures required. Also mineral residues remain dissolved during wet oxidation.

I emphasize the need for a "good" oxidation method. Many times just getting the material into solution is thought to be an acceptable solution for analysis. There is grave danger that much of the organic matter is still in solution and not oxidized. Particulate matter contains much of the material that is needed for a complete analysis.

There are advantages and disadvantages to both methods of analysis. XRF is not capable, with our present system, to analyze for the lighter elements such as Mg, Na, K, Li or the metals Cd and Mo.

Using the ICP type of analysis, these elements can be detected, the source of error here being loss of particular "volatile elements" in the oxidation procedure.

MINERAL PATTERNS AND DISEASE STATES    The medical anecdote is not to be overlooked in a field in its infancy. The following article, by Jack Challem, was printed for Biochemical Concepts Laboratory, Albuquerque, New Mexico, and released to nutritionists. While not "scientific" in the sense of double-blind studies, the anecdotal cases cited are worthy of our interest. Properly employed, hair analysis patterns and corrective diets may hold promise in treating arthritis, adult onset diabetes, high blood pressure, fatigue, chronic lower back pain, and rheumatoid arthritis, as well as toxicity states from lead, cadmium, aluminum, and mercury.

Bill Russell, who is also a Medical Technologist and Clinical Toxicologist, offered the interesting case history of his mother and how hair analysis helped her health. According to Russell, his mother had suffered from arthritis and nodules on her fingers. "The hair analysis showed her to have a typical arthritic pattern: high calcium, low magnesium and low manganese. A high level of calcium in the hair shows that the calcium is not where it should be metabolically. She was placed on a diet low in refined carbohydrates, and was given supplements of B-complex vitamins, magnesium, manganese, and Vitamin E. In three weeks she received relief from the aching in her hands. In eight weeks her fingers stopped locking. Slowly, over a period of a year, the nodules on her fingers are decreasing. She continues to take the magnesium, B-complex and E."

In addition to analyzing the evaluating mineral levels in the hair of individuals, Bill Russell and his associate Charles Puckett, Technical Director of Biochemical Concepts Laboratory, have correlated relationships between particular mineral patterns and disease states.

Their medical director, Charles Rudolph, Jr., reported on some of their results in the July, 1977, issue of the *Journal of the International Academy of Preventive Medicine*. In this paper, "Trace Element Patterning in Degenerative Diseases," Dr. Rudolph noted that persons with adult onset diabetes have a critical nutrition problem in that they are characteristically low in magnesium, zinc, chromium and manganese of which the latter three compose the *Glucose Tolerance Factor* (a chemical necessary to properly metabolize sugars).

With regard to high blood pressure, a very common condition in the United States, Dr. Rudolph pointed out that the "most significant finding in the hypertensive individuals is that of increased cellular cadmium levels. . . . Cadmium has a very potent hypertensive effect at low levels in the tissues." Cadmium antagonizes the essential mineral zinc, interfering with normal zinc metabolism and the sixty-odd enzyme reactions in which zinc is involved.

In fatigue of "undetermined origin" two toxic elements, cadmium and lead, are found elevated. In cases of nervousness and anxiety, the trend seems to be low levels of manganese and magnesium.

With regard to chronic low back discomfort, the pattern seems to be low potassium levels. "Low tissue potassium may predispose to muscle fatigability, the probable origin of the low back discomfort."

Patients with rheumatoid arthritis demonstrate elevated levels of lead. Lead, according to Rudolph, "stimulates the enzyme hyaluronidase, which in turn stimulates the breakdown of hyaluronic acid, a component of the joint lubricating fluid." It might be added that the most common source of lead in the environment comes from gasoline to which the metal is added as an antiknock compound.

Used preventively by persons in good health, hair analysis might point out tendencies toward particular disease conditions which might not reveal themselves in symptoms for years to come. With the knowledge thus gained it becomes very easy to prevent such conditions from arising.

*Arthritis, Diabetes, Fatigue, Back Pain, May Be Related to Trace Mineral Status*

In terms of diagnosing diseases already present, mineral levels in the hair are fairly representative of stores in the body. Interpreted along with the constituents of the patient's diet a physician familiar with this procedure can determine whether high levels of certain minerals may be due to loss from the body, or from turn-over of excesses. Similarly, low levels of minerals in the hair may indicate low tissue levels throughout the body, poor absorption or some other difficulty.

To detect potentially chronic micronutrient dietary deficiencies, hair analysis offers an accurate, non-invasive method of analyzing the body's mineral make-up. Used in conjuction with a practical knowledge of the mineral content of foods, hair analysis can be useful as a diagnostic tool and serves as an aid in helping to maintain or regain a healthy body.*

On a preventive level, hair analysis should be a part of every nutritional analysis, if only to determine levels of toxic metals. Elevated levels of metals such as lead, cadmium, mercury, and aluminum do *not* reflect individual needs *or* ethnic differences; they are obviously a reflection of environmental exposure (air, water, food, tobacco, certain alcoholic drinks, etc.), and must be seen as extremely important values for any proper nutritional workup.

---

* Unfortunately, at this time hair analysis is useful only in determining levels of toxic metals.

Better is a dry morsel and quietness therewith than a house of feasting with strife.

—PROVERBS 17:1

# 13
# A STRATEGY FOR DAILY DINING

Healthy people without allergies to specific foods (such as milk and dairy, gluten, sucrose, and other dietary items already discussed) can easily calculate their own nutritional program. Having read to this point, we can accept the following dietary coordinates:

1. Eat only when hungry.
2. Drink only when thirsty.
3. Elimination should never be neglected, not for a moment!
4. No food should be taken without first warming the body to a roseate glow, by walking or other light exercise.
5. The stomach should be one-quarter full at breakfast, three-quarters full at lunch, and one-half full at supper.
6. Reduce fats and oils eaten by 15 percent.
7. Reduce sugar and syrup intake to near 0 percent (eat fruit).
8. Reduce meat intake by 20 percent; increase consumption of fish and poultry accordingly.
9. Increase amount of potatoes eaten (by 15 percent); other vegetables (by 15 percent); fruit (by 15 percent); and whole grains. Snack on nuts.
10. Reduce milk and dairy consumption by 10 percent; eat a maximum of four eggs per week.
11. Reduce use of alcoholic drinks; shift to wine and beer.
12. Throw away the salt shaker (adequate salt is found naturally in most foods).
13. Balance your inner chemistry; 60 percent alkaline/40 percent acid-forming foods.
14. Avoid highly processed foods and those with chemical additives.

While dietary specifics will vary depending upon culture, geographical niche, and individual preferences, the above rules will prove valuable for most people living in America and Western Europe. Ethnic diets can be modified to meet these dietary goals without losing their unique properties. But remember, what we now consider to be a typical Italian, Jewish, Chinese, Greek, Mexican, or other "ethnic" meal is atypical. Based upon available evidence, most meals now eaten in ethnic restaurants are more like feasts than authentic daily fare. People go "out to eat" festively on a daily basis, with consequent health problems, largely due to overeating. Reinforcing what Maimonides, the wise twelfth-century physician, has written: "Over-eating is like a deadly poison to any constitution and is the principal cause of all diseases. Most maladies that afflict mankind result from bad food or are due to the patient filling his stomach with an excess of food that may even have been wholesome."

Our difficulty stems from the complex stresses that surround us; we tend to lose contact with our inner selves, so that we are no longer able to respond to the subtle cues that tell us when we are hungry or satiated. We generally eat three meals a day whether we are hungry or not. The clock tells us when to eat, not our inner selves. The food is piled on our plates. We are told it is "sinful and wasteful" not to consume everything, so our plates are cleaned, and it is only correct and polite that our plates be filled to the maximum. Instead of ceasing well before we are full, we consume everything, rising from the table complaining of distress with a smile on our face, and complaining how our abdomen feels tight and hurts and how we are virtually nauseated. What a marvelous state to be in, when food is supposed to be giving us pleasure! Instead we have learned to interpret discomfort as pleasure!

The "strategy for daily dining" approach allows for individual differences, but to understand certain of the fourteen principles we should realize that an "optimal diet" will differ according to ethnic, genetic, or energy levels. For example, the daily activity level of an African Bushman is quite different from that of an urban New Yorker. These differences in *lifestyle* by themselves would significantly modify the needs for an optimal diet. The African Bushman is usually smaller, thinner, and much more active than the New York urbanite, who is usually larger and, until recently at least, extremely sedentary. Further, contemporary urban dwellers generally consume a considerable amount of alcohol, as may the African Bushman from time to time, but not on so regular a basis. The African Bushman collects and utilizes foodstuffs within his ecological niche, eating from a relatively *wide* variety of materials, whereas the urbanite, who believes that he has available all the world's foods and foodstuffs, in reality is eating from an extremely *limited* variety of foods (combined and packaged in almost limitless ways).

And so, to compute our own dietary needs we must also evaluate factors such as our energy requirements as well.

# Using the Computerized Dietary Analysis

When calculating our protein, carbohydrate, fat, vitamin, and mineral intake from the foods we eat (using a computer-generated nutrition-analysis form), we will want to compare how much of each nutrient we are getting with the RDAs.

A sample dietary analysis might look like this:

## *Nutrition, Health, and Activity Profile\**

OF HAROLD SMITH

C/O DR. MICHAEL WEINER

SUMMARY OF 5/7/79    AGE 47    WT 210    SEX M

| | Daily Intake | Recommended Intake |
|---|---|---|
| Weekly Exercise Calories: 2538 | | |
| Total calories | 3,270 | |
| Protein (grams) | 122.2 | 85.1–108 |
| Fat (grams) | 145.8 | |
| Calories from fat | 1,312 | |
| Percent calories from fat | 40.1 | 20–34 |
| Linoleic acid (grams) | 24.2 | 3–5 |
| Fiber (grams) | 14.6 | 6 |
| Carbohydrates (grams) | 379.6[1] | |
| Refined (grams) | 20.5[2] | |
| Percent refined | 5[3] | |

[1] Calories: 1454; percent calories: 44.
[2] Equals 5 tsp sugar.
[3] Including alcohol: 8 percent.
\* Courtesy of Pacific Research Systems, Los Angeles, California.

| Vitamins | COL. 1<br>Daily<br>Intake | COL. 2<br>U.S.<br>RDA | COL. 3<br>Percent of<br>RDA | COL. 4<br>Currently<br>Takes This<br>Vitamin |
|---|---|---|---|---|
| Vitamin A (IU) | 15,635 | 5,000 | 312.7 | Yes |
| Vitamin C (mg) | 505.1 | 60 | 841.8 | Yes |
| Vitamin E (IU) | 7.8 | 30 | 25.9 | Yes |
| Vitamin B$_1$ (mg)—Thiamine | 3.7 | 1.5 | 243.5 | Yes |
| Vitamin B$_2$ (mg)—Riboflavin | 1.9 | 1.7 | 111.2 | Yes |
| Vitamin B$_3$ (mg)—Niacin | 33.5 | 20 | 167.6 | Yes |
| Vitamin B$_6$ (mg)—Pyridoxine | 3.7 | 2 | 185.9 | Yes |
| Folacin (mg)—Folic acid | 224 | 400 | 56.1 | Yes |
| Vitamin B$_{12}$ (mg) | 7.2 | 6 | 120.2 | Yes |
| Pantothenic Acid (mg) | 9.5 | 10 | 95.1 | Yes |
| Biotin (mg) | 102 | 300 | 34 | Yes |
| Choline (mg) | 642 | — | — | |
| Inositol (mg) | 1,570 | — | — | |

| Minerals | Daily<br>Intake | U.S.<br>RDA | Percent of<br>RDA | Currently<br>Takes This<br>Mineral |
|---|---|---|---|---|
| Calcium (mg) | 903[1] | 1,000 | 90.3 | Yes |
| Phosphorus (mg) | 2,987[1] | 1,000 | 298.7 | Yes |
| Magnesium (mg) | 511 | 400 | 127.9 | Yes |
| Iron (mg) | 24.9 | 18 | 138.1 | Yes |
| Copper (mg) | 0.5 | 2 | 25.6 | Yes |
| Zinc (mg) | 8.3 | 15 | 55.1 | Yes |
| Iodine (mg) in food only | 66 | 150 | 44.3 | Yes |
| Manganese (mg) | 1.6 | — | — | [2] |
| Potassium (mg) | 6,409 | — | — | [2] |
| Sodium (mg) in food only | 2,362 | — | — | [2] |
| Fluorine (mg) | 999 | — | — | [2] |

HEALTH FACTORS:
1. Diabetes in family
2. Takes drugs regularly
3. High blood pressure
4. Drinks tap water

[1] Calcium and phosphorus are out of balance.
[2] Has taken supplements for more than 1 year.

Looking at the first entry, we see that this client burns off 2,538 calories weekly from exercising. Of course, by performing daily acts such as sitting, walking, writing, driving, and so on, he also uses calories. Harold Smith's protein intake is 122.2 grams daily, and looking to the right, we see that a recommended intake (varying according to expert opinion) ranges from between 85.1 to 108 grams of protein daily, a reduction of about 10 to 25 percent.

The fat Harold eats accounts for 40.1 percent of his overall food intake, while a reduction to between 20 to 34 percent fats in his daily diet is urged, in this age of cancer. Surprisingly, we learn that Mr. Smith is somehow taking in 24.2 grams of linoleic acid, when only 3 to 5 grams are recommended. A typical Western diet is very low in this fatty acid, essential for promoting the production of prostaglandin, and also stimulating the immune system in other ways (see Horrobin, 1979). To get your 3 to 5 grams of linoleic acid you need to take only one tablespoonsful of soy, corn, peanut, safflower, or sunflower seed oil, usually as salad dressing or for stir-frying your meals.

Harold's fiber intake, 14.6 grams, is well above the 6 grams minimally required, and leagues beyond the 2 to 3 grams contained in an average refined-carbohydrate, low-vegetable-and-fruit diet. Mr. Smith eats all of his fruits in the fresh state, and generally prefers his vegetables raw, another wise food choice.

Carbohydrate intake, which accounts for 44 percent of total calories, would not be too great if they were complex carbohydrates (whole grains, potatoes, fruits, and vegetables, etc.). But here we see that Mr. Smith takes in 20.5 grams of *refined* carbohydrate (of 5 percent of his total carbohydrate intake). This is not bad, a fact reflecting the patient's dietary adjustment of a year ago, when he changed his eating patterns to include more whole foods, including whole-wheat bread. Diabetes is in his family history and Harold has acted wisely by restricting the sugars, syrups, white bread, pasta, pastries, and cookies.

To gain some perspective on the amount of carbohydrates eaten, bear in mind that the average citizen in the United States eats about 120 pounds of refined sweetener per year. This is thirty times more than the average colonist ate in the year 1700. One group of consumer-oriented nutritionists calculated that this amount of refined sweetener equals about 720 apple pies per person per year; but remember, sugar is found not only in the raw form or in the purified form, but it also appears

in many breakfeast cereals, pies, pastries, snacks, canned vegetables, canned fish, baby food. As a purified food without any
nutrients other than energy, sugar seems to disturb normal
carbohydrate nutrition, and according to Yudkin (1972) it is
largely responsible for many cases of diabetes and heart disease.
The sugar habit can easily be broken, simply by switching to
fresh fruits, particularly bananas, when hungry for a sweet.
Dates and raisins are also available, as are other sweet fruits.
Here we receive natural sugars associated with many vitamins
and minerals also present in fruit, and the all-important dietary
fiber.

In the first years of this century, when diets were much
closer to those of Europe, the average person in the United
States consumed about 225 pounds of flour, half of which were
whole wheat. By 1976 only 111 pounds of flour were eaten by
the average person, and astoundingly 104 pounds of this consisted of refined white flour, which contains only 8 percent of
the fiber found in whole wheat. Likewise, in the last fifty years
the amount of fresh fruits and vegetables, also consisting of
complex carbohydrates and fiber, vitamins and minerals, has
fallen by well over 50 percent, with an increased consumption
of processed vegetables and fruits, with much sugar in the pack-
aging. To reverse this trend, both Mr. Smith and the average
person in developed nations must eat more like his ancestors
of fifty or sixty years ago, with a greater emphasis upon whole-
grain flours, more fruits and vegetables, less meat, less protein,
less fat, less salt, and by far fewer additives and preservatives.

Looking now at Mr. Smith's vitamin intake from foods
alone, we see in Column 1 that his vitamin A intake is 15,635
IU. In Column 2 we note that the U.S. RDA is 5,000 units.
In Column 3 we see that Mr. Smith is receiving 312.7 percent
of the RDA; that is, from foods alone he receives well over
three times the amount of vitamin A recommended by the
Food and Nutrition Board. In the case of this vitamin, this
is certainly wise, because while it is certainly fat soluble and
toxic at very high dosage, the figure set for the RDA, that
is, 5,000 IU per day, is, like all other figures in Column 2,
merely a subsistence level.

Briefly reviewing the list, we see that Mr. Smith receives
505.1 mg of vitamin C a day, when the RDA is only 60 mg,
which accounts for the figure of 841.8 percent of the RDA in
Column 3. Again, this is owing to the large amount of fresh
fruits and vegetables in Mr. Smith's diet. Notice, though, that
even this man who is wise enough to consume so many fruits

and vegetables is highly deficient in vitamin E. He receives only 7.8 IU a day, when the RDA, an already low figure, calls for 30 units a day; and so in Column 3 we notice that he receives only 25.9 percent of the vitamin E required.

Looking down the column, we see that he receives adequate or more than adequate amounts of vitamins $B_1$, $B_2$, $B_3$, and $B_6$, but that his intake of folic acid is only 56.1 percent of the RDA. Further down, we see that his pantothenic acid intake is 95.1 percent of the recommended daily allowance, and that his biotin intake is only 34 percent. His daily intake of choline and inositol are given, while Column 2 contains no recommended amount, and of course therefore Column 3 doesn't list a percent of the RDA. To find out the function of inositol, choline, biotin, all of the other vitamins and minerals, please refer to an earlier chapter, "Overcoming the Famine Within." This excellent synopsis also gives common food sources of the various vitamins and minerals, which is certainly the preferred way to make up for any deficiencies that may appear when computing your own dietary needs.

Looking at Mr. Smith's intake of calcium, we notice he takes in 903 mg a day, when his phosphorus is highly elevated, a typical American pattern, at near 3,000 mg a day. Thus his phosphorus intake is three times that of calcium, when the RDAs indicate that they should be equal to each other. Calcium and phosphorus are out of balance, as noted in the computerized report. This imbalance is typical of diets that emphasize beef, chicken, and fish, which are all generally phosphorus rich and not too high in calcium. Our primitive ancestors were in better balance because they ate the bones in addition to the meat. This is why cracking chicken bones and eating the ends is a good idea, as is gnawing on any bone when you are eating the meat. Of course, phosphorus levels vary in different types of meats. For example, beef liver contains 352 mg of phosphorus per 100 grams, while beef steak contains 142 mg of phosphorus. Rabbit, now in demand owing to its low cholesterol levels, is one of the highest phosphorus-containing meats, at 352 mg per 100 grams. All cuts of lamb are comparatively lower in phosphorus, ranging between 125 and 150 mg per 100 grams. Tripe, a very popular dish in certain ethnic menus, contains 127 mg of calcium and only 86 mg of phosphorus, one of the few animal foods with a positive calcium to phosphorus balance.

Just as various meats differ in their calcium and phosphorus ratios, this is also true with fish. For example, crabmeat contains

43 mg of calcium and 175 mg of phosphorus per 100 grams of edible material, while oysters contain 94 mg calcium and 143 mg of phosphorus. Salmon contains 79 mg calcium and 186 mg of phosphorus, while swordfish contains only 19 mg of calcium and 195 mg of phosphorus. One of the highest known phosphorus levels in fish is found in shad, which contains 260 mg of phosphorus and 20 mg of calcium.

A wise rule to keep in mind while working with your dietary preferences is to increase calcium-rich foods while decreasing those foods with high phosphorus contents.

Continuing with Mr. Smith's computerized dietary form, we notice that his intake of copper at 0.5 mg is only 25.6 percent of the recommended level of 2 mg per day. Next to that we see that his intake of zinc is also low, being only 55.1 percent of an already too low 15 mg of the RDA. Further, his iodine intake, as is typical in most Western diets, is only 44.3 percent of the RDA.

# Nutritional Dispensation

While many people come to see me for nutritional dispensation—that is, they pay me to forgive them for their dietary excesses—most people find it useful to have a computerized analysis of their daily food intake and also a hair analysis. By looking at the results of both forms, we can then devise an optimum diet for most people, without resorting to pre-printed diets but by concentrating on foods that are particularly rich in nutrients the client may be deficient in, and by more or less staying with foods that people have adapted to and seem to prefer. A painless shift to wiser, more adaptive diets is easily effected.

# Fasting

*Fasting*
*Adaptive*

Abstaining from food and drink for limited intervals has been part of every major religion since antiquity and appears to offer the follower a sense of self-discipline that is beneficial. Of course, such fasting also served (and continues to serve) as a wise means of conserving food supplies. In a country like India, a thirty-day limited fast is part of the annual cycle and serves as a means of reducing the overall food needs of a vast population.

Certainly, *limiting* the intake of food is advisable in a land of plenty, but fasting per se is a matter of individual choice, not something to be undertaken on a regular basis and recommended for everybody. Hypoglycemic people, for instance, often experience dangerously low blood sugar levels during even limited fasts. For these individuals lengthy abstinence from food and drink often brings a return of symptoms, sometimes with alarming results.*

*Hypoglycemics Advised Not to Fast*

For healthy people who want an occasional fast (to shrink their stomach, rest their digestive tract and kidneys, and otherwise "slow down"), a short fast (two to three days) is recommended. *Total* fasting is not wise, owing to the physiological stress that results from starvation.

After three to four days of starvation (or total fasting), ketosis and a mild metabolic acidosis progress, with "a gradual and continued excretion of calcium and phosphorus in amounts beyond that lost from the lean tissue being catabolized." Bone mineral is slowly dissolved (!), making "some clinicians reluctant to use starvation or ketogenic diets in individuals prone to osteoporosis, such as Caucasian females" (Cahill, 1978).

*Ketosis and Acidosis Result from Long Fasts*

Other negative results of lengthy, total fasts include a rise in serum urate levels and, rarely, liver enlargement, particularly in people who have previously had a liver disease such as hepatitis. The physiology of fasting is an interesting topic discussed by Cahill, but not possible here. But I will include one final comment, again from Cahill's interesting study:

*Uric Acid Level Rises*

Vitamins are probably unnecessary with total starvation, the need for the B vitamins, particularly $B_1$ and for vitamin C occurring only when carbohydrates are eaten. The Arctic explorer died with scurvy and beriberi eating his crackers while his Eskimo guide survived on blubber.

## A Cleansing Fast** (3 days only)

JUICE FAST NO. 1

3 Day:  Mix sweet juices (pear, apple, pineapple) 50/50 with water, all other fruits available at full strength. Alternate the different fruits throughout the day in order to get a good variety each day.

* The sudden exacerbation of hypoglycemia, in an individual who has stabilized her condition through careful dietary adjustment, can bring about a suicidal depression.

** Devised by Anabolic Foods, Irvine, California.

Green Drink: 75% carrot juice, 15% celery, 10% mixed leafy green vegetables (any edible green leaf vegetable). Change the 10% mixed leafy green vegetables for each 8 oz of juice such as 10% spinach, etc. In some 8 oz use 5% parsley and 5% green peppers as the 10%.

7:00 A.M.:   Fruit juice 8 oz

9:00 A.M.:   Green drink 8 oz

11:00 A.M.:   Fruit juice 8 oz

1:00 P.M.:   Green drink 8 oz

3:00 P.M.:   Fruit juice 8 oz

5:00 P.M.:   Green drink 8 oz

7:00 P.M.:   Vegetable broth 8 oz

9:00 P.M.:   Vegetable broth 8 oz

Be sure juice and broth are made fresh each day.

## Vegetable Broth Recipe

2 large potatoes, unpeeled, chopped or sliced to ½-inch pieces

1 cup carrots, shredded or sliced

1 cup red beets, shredded or sliced

1 cup celery, leaves and all, chopped to ½-inch pieces

1 cup any other available vegetable: beet tops, turnips and turnip tops, parsley, cabbage, etc.

Use stainless steel, enameled, or earthenware utensil. Fill it up with one and one-half quarts of water and slice the vegetables directly into the water to prevent oxidation. Cover and cook slowly for 30 minutes. Let stand for another 30 minutes; strain; cool until warm and serve or refrigerate.

# 14 "THE DIETARY DEBATE OF THE CENTURY": ATKINS VS. PRITIKIN

Any genuine ethnic cookbook can be reinterpreted to incorporate a reduced consumption of butter and other animal fats, salt, sugar and refined carbohydrates, and additives, while increasing the amount of whole foods, i.e., brown rice, whole wheat, fresh vegetables and fruits, raw honey, and cold-pressed vegetable oils. In this sense, recipes are unnecessary. We all have our dietary likes and dislikes—we need only adjust the relative proportions in the plate (*less* protein, *less* fat, *more* unrefined carbohydrate) and buy purer raw materials to eat as we choose.

Yet diet books abound, so there is some need for "menus" in the Western mind. Cookbooks, as any competent chef will tell you, are to be avoided, as are the extreme menus of dietary messiahs. Nutrition as a science reappears before us at a time when the growing spirit of eclecticism encourages many intelligent and skeptically sound people to listen to, and even try, all new doctrines with an alacrity liable to degenerate into weakness. In the context of the present exploration of diverse diets, the concept of "scientific nutrition" is sometimes alluded to, but its specific precepts are little known and unclearly comprehended. This is understandable in light of the relative lack of nutrition education among most diet-book writers.

## "The Debate of the Century"

At a recent conference of the Orthomolecular Medical Society, the "debate of the century" between Atkins and Pritikin was more of a personality contest than an exposition of scientific evidence.

*Opposite Positions Offered as the Truth*

As Atkins, the self-assured, cosmopolitan, slightly plump physician spoke, I was cajoled into relaxing my strict low-fat grasp on reality, no longer fearing an immediate heart attack if I chose to eat a steak. His "evidence" for the efficacy of his high-fat, high-protein, low-carbohydrate diet consisted of a glib manner, an engaging charm, and an apparent total lack of preparedness for this contest.

Pritikin, the thin health-entrepreneur, appeared to be better equipped for the debate, with superbly crafted charts and tables.

*Author Fears for His Life*

I don't recall the exact approach employed, but as this debate went on I became increasingly paranoid about my cardiac risk profile until I was positively sweating with anxiety by the time the lights were raised. He managed to convince me that Atkins was completely wrong and that only *his* high-carbohydrate, low-protein, near-zero-fat diet was medically wise. I was so hypnotized by the cadence of blue slides that I became certain my very life had been threatened by a few olives, my daily wine, and the occasional lamb shank I had allowed myself!

*Why Pay to Starve?*

After the polite applause, the actual debate began, with Atkins accusing his opponent of being "more concerned with the longevity of the Longevity Institute [Pritikin's creation] than with the longevity of his clients." This was a low blow, but rather funny, especially when you consider how many thousands of dollars people pay to eat diets similar to African beekeepers, who have little choice but to subsist on grains, fruit, and grubs! I myself wondered why anybody needed to *pay* to starve themselves. But then, my skepticism has never made it easy for me to sit very well at academic congresses.

*Pritikin Diet Not Right for All People*

The "Pritikin Diet" is a new version of previous high-carbohydrate diets. This diet recommends that you eat 80 percent carbohydrate (unrefined), 10–15 percent protein, and 5–10 percent fat. The typical American diet, by comparison, consists of 45 percent carbohydrate (largely refined), 10–20 percent protein, and 40–45 percent fat. In addition, you are required to abstain from alcohol, caffeine, cigarettes, and to exercise extensively.

Now I have no qualms with those who like this sort of monotony. But the evidence that this regimen will reduce the symptoms of angina pectoris, reduce serum cholesterol, uric acid levels, and triglycerides and enable you to give up antihypertensive drugs, insulin, and oral hypoglycemic agents is merely claimed, not substantiated by any long-term studies. Sure, it makes sense that we reverse our overdependence on fats and refined carbohydrates, but to prescribe this for everyone is precisely the "food fascism" I disavowed in Chapter 1.

On a strictly scientific level the "Pritikin Diet" is also wrong for individuals with increased nutrient requirements—such people as growing children; pregnant and lactating women; and those with infections, chronic illnesses, or those suffering from malnutrition. In addition, any high-carbohydrate, low-fat diet creates special problems in these areas: linoleic acid, an important component of the "auto-immune complex" defined by Dr. Horrobin, may be deficient when you restrict fats to the degree suggested by Pritikin; as we have seen, phytates, a component of whole grains, may limit the absorption of minerals such as calcium and zinc and of trace metals such as molybdenum and chromium; and the iron supplied in this diet is largely from "non-heme" sources, and is less well absorbed than iron from "heme" sources found in animal products. Finally, referring again to our discussion of diet and coronary heart disease, the study in India by Malhotra (1967) showed us that northern Indians, who are avid eaters of milk products and ghee, rich in saturated fatty-acids, suffer from less than one-fifteenth the number of heart attacks that occur in a group of southern Indians of the same occupation who are vegetarians and consume diets with only 2 percent saturated fats. This, we saw, may be due to the fact that "the butter fat and fermented-milk drinks common to the northern Indians promote the intestinal flora and presumably the intestinal synthesis of pyridoxine, while the unsaturated fats of the southern Indians need to be accompanied by more pyridoxine in the diet, depress intestinal flora synthesis, and depress calcium absorption." (Williams, 1973).

Like jogging, such an extremely restricted diet is an over-reaction to overly rich foods. Why not a balanced reaction, and a moderately revised diet? Americans, it seems, like extremes. First, we are the most sedentary people on Earth. Now we are the most hyperactive inhabitants, running everywhere to the detriment of our poor tendons, knees, and without clear benefit to our hearts! Walking will do, as will a rational diet based on the principles outlined in this book and summarized on page 215, "A Strategy for Daily Dining." *Diet Extremes Likened to Jogging*

Of course, my view is largely based on anecdotal evidence, but since the messianic leaders themselves offer little more than anecdotal data which they each use to convince us of their wisdom, I introduce *my* bias in an attempt to disavow the *Readers Urged to Devise Their Own Diet* craving for a benevolent nutrition-czar among millions of floundering people. To truly arrive at a reasonable diet for yourself *you* must do the necessary work—read the ancients and the theories, perhaps order a computerized dietary analysis, and then outline your own nutritional program—which incorporates your food preferences and abhorences, reasonably and without anxiety.

*Disquieting Doubts Not Undoubted Truths*

And so, I now leave you to your own decision. If either of the two examined dietary schools (the mono-medical school of "eat as you will," the holistic school of "eat only what I say"), "shall upon rational and experimental grounds be clearly made out to me, 'tis obliging, but not irrational, in you to expect, that I shall not be so farr in love with my disquieting doubts, as not to be content to change them for undoubted truths." And though I be an irresolute skeptic I will confess that as unsatisfied as I appear to be with the doctrines current in nutrition, be they mono-medical or holistic, "I can yet so little discover what to acquiesce in, that perchance the enquiries of others have scarce been more unsatisfactory to me, than my own have been to myself" (Boyle, 1680).

# 15
# HOLISTIC HEALTH:
# A HAVEN IN DEMISE?

*Illness as Recreation*

Recreational illness, having been spurred in part by a new leisure enjoyed through all classes of society, may account for *some* part of the contemporary search for medical alternatives. But our growing discontent with the high costs and continually unfolding dangers of modern medicine are *real.* We now spend proportionately more of our money on doctors and medicines than in the past, while documented cases of iatrogenic disorders also escalate. People are questioning the necessity of the massive drugging with synthetic compounds, the almost knee-jerk ordering of diagnostic and surgical techniques, and the loss of a personal touch from the physician-healer.

Just as environmentalists advocate the nondisruption of our ecology, so do alternative health theorists profess to treat illness with minimal disruption of the body's internal environment. Medical systems that have been employed in other culture for hundreds, even thousands, of years, such as the Chinese system of acupuncture, are now offered by the new students of alternative healing.

*Medical "Alternatives" Questioned*

This great interest in and practice of alternative medicine is also driven by the notion that the medical establishment is more mercenary than you and I. But how can we be certain that alternative health practitioners are themselves not guilty of this motive? Certainly the fee schedules are not much lower than those levied by licensed, educated health professionals. Too many "alternative healers" have undertaken little if any serious study. In fact, many self-styled doctors in America have simply read one or two popular books and then gone on to prescribe, treating people for every kind of infirmity from halitosis to cancer. Are we to believe that these people are divinely inspired, that precisely because they are uneducated they have a secret design for methods of healing unknown to licensed, educated professionals.?

This is not to argue that medicine as we now know it and all licensed practitioners are the epitome of a health-care system. I have chosen to criticize the New Wave medicine because of elements within the movement which offer no alternative to the existing exploitative currents, while pretending to do so.

*The Author's Position Likened to Boyle's*

Like Boyle, who achieved immediate success with his book *The Sceptical Chymist* by ridiculing two opposing schools (the four elements of the philosophers and the three elements of the alchemists who professed occult qualities in natural objects), I stand between the old-guard medical practitioners who maintain that, except in rare instances, the dietary treatment of disease per se is virtually a myth, and the holistic practitioners who apparently see in every inner disharmony and all diseases a dietary relationship.

## My Battle

*Diet* Not *Our Salvation*

Existing somewhere between the two schools described above, I insist that diet is related to disease and health, in the main, but we must not look to food as our salvation, nor seek to soothe all inner disharmonies that are a part of life on this planet. Going beyond food, nutrition, and health, the same concepts apply to the entire spectrum of illness and medicine. We must not rush toward a concept of health that is selfish to the exclusion of everyone but our own little needs. Many of us have a tendency toward being that "self-centered little clod of ailments and grievances" described by George Bernard Shaw. Before embracing a system of medicine and healing that tends to amplify this selfishness, we must correct direction, incorporating the best elements from the world's principal healing systems.

## The Need for Prohibition: An Ancient Theme

In biblical times the priests acted as guardians of public health while physicians were also considered to be endowed with spiritual powers. God was seen as the only healer, the physicians revered as the helpers or instruments of Divine authority.

Specific dietary prohibitions of the Hebrew Scriptures have shaped and influenced Christian civilization to a degree not previously recognized. Among the early Hebrews, man was told for the first time what *not* to eat at the risk of offending the Creator and suffering the dreaded consequences.

While Christian peoples enjoy a freedom from the severe dietary retraints of Orthodox Judaism, there lurks a faint memory of certain foods, namely pork and shellfish, as forbidden. While many other categories of edibles are prohibited in the Orthodox Jewish world, most Christians seem to maintain a vague remembrance of these Jewish food prohibitions.

*Jewish Food Prohibitions Lay Groundwork*

During epidemics disease was often regarded as Divine retribution for transgressions. Thus until recently most of mankind looked toward heaven and the spirits when a health disaster fell upon them. In these times, when heart disease and cancer are epidemics of historical significance, something faint in us still believes that if only we were a little better spiritually our physical entities would not be plagued by these diseases. We know carcinogens exist, just as we are all convinced by now that smoking cigarettes, becoming sluggish, emphasizing the lipids and sugars, all contribute to our cardiac risk profile.

But in the back of our minds we want an authority to tell us these things—no, to go further and admonish us for our easy ways, prescribing and proscribing what is fit and what is foul, both in diet and activities.

# Enter the Alternative Practitioner

As we grew more lax, so did our mainstream physicians. They were just as subject to disease as the general population, often *looked* downright unhealthy (in biblical days a mere blemish would disqualify a man from serving as a priest!); many smoked, even while treating us, and the psychiatrists—well, it became disturbing to learn that they enjoyed the highest of suicide rates.

The New Age "healers," on the other hand, presented a more acceptable image. They were generally lean, younger, nonsmokers, often female. With an array of healing techniques spanning centuries and of great repute, an irresistible appeal created an inexhaustible patient load. At last we thought we could enjoy pain-free, joyful existences, without the dangers of X rays, costly laboratory examinations, synthetic drugs, and all the other entrapments of high-tech medicine. Our new healers were supposed to be more feeling, more sensitive—in short, more healing; and all this was thought to come at prices far below medical norms.

*Holistic Healers Fulfilled Our Need for Admonishment*

Often these healers gave advice that satisfied our needs to do without! Many of us were told to give up all dairy products by the acupuncturist, schooled in an ancient Asian medical system that evolved *without* milk and milk products. In fact, the Chinese who invented acupuncture (about five thousand years ago) rejected dairy products with loathing at that time. This was due to the limited number of dairy-producing animals in ancient China, and also because other Asian cultural groups—Indians, Tibetans, and central Asian nomads—depended on milk so heavily.

*Milk and Dairy Rejected*

These cultural barriers broke down in time, allowing an intermingling of food beliefs. After Han times (206 B.C.–A.D. 220), Chinese and Altaic customs intermixed and concurrently the prejudice against milk diminished. By T'ang times (A.D. 618) milk products were enjoyed by all upper-class Chinese on a regular basis. In north China goat's milk was considered of value to the kidneys, by the time of this dynasty, while in the south carabao milk formed a part of many popular dishes. From Iran came a famed sweet, "stone honey," made of water buffalo milk and sugar.

Nevertheless, during the period when acupuncture was *first* developed, milk products were loathed in China, and this loathing may have been carried wholesale by Western acupuncturists and Oriental healers.

This is not to say that the restriction of dairy products is not wise for some people. The point is that the wholesale rejection of this class of foods may be based upon outmoded concepts of health. The reason giving up dairy products often brings about relief from sinus conditions and other allergic-type conditions may be more the result of decreasing the intake of antibiotics and hormones found in milk than from any inherent nutritive substances (said to be "mucous forming"). The alternative practitioner and holistic physician should consider suggesting "raw" (i.e., nonhomogenized) dairy products derived from animals raised on drug-free diets. These foods are available, and provide a good source of calcium and other constituents necessary for growth.

If further argument is required to convince our dairy prohibitionists of the nutritional values of this important human food, antiquity is a ready reference.

Both Isaiah, the Hebrew prophet, and a prominent Indian educator share a belief in milk and honey as an elixir—a belief of ancient origin found in several dissimilar cultures:

Curd and honey shall he eat, when he knoweth to refuse the evil, and choose the good.

—ISAIAH 7:15

Omar V. Garrison, a scholar of Tantric yoga, reports the words of an Indian, Pundit Chatterjee, who recommends a recipe for long life similar to Isaiah's: a mixture containing a fat-rich dairy product:

If you were to ask me to single out one food that, more than any other, is a Tantrik food, then I would say at once: honey. Mix it with ghee (clarified butter) in the proportion of three to one and take a tablespoonful morning and evening. Some years ago, the newspapers both here and abroad carried an account concerning Srijut Malaviya, one of our prominent educators, who had discovered some secret of rejuvenation. It was reported that he had turned back the clock twenty years, so far as his personal appearance and vitality were concerned.

I journeyed to Benares for the express purpose of learning from his own lips how he had accomplished it. When I pressed him for details, he told me that the chief dietary item in his remarkable discipline was honey mixed with ghee. (Garrison, 1964)

Experts on *Food in Antiquity,* the Brothwells believe "that milking was early established in Neolithic communities," adding that cow and goat milk were the type most generally used in ancient communities. The Greeks, we learn, preferred the milk from goats and sheep in diluted form, while Pliny notes that the sweetest milk comes from the camel. Sarmatian tribes had an interesting dairy-based recipe: "millet meal with mare's milk or with blood from a horse's leg vein." Other ancient peoples left records of their likings for milk from reindeer, elk, yaks, and asses.

*Dairy Products Greatly Valued in Antiquity*

Milk products such as butter, cheese, and sour milk are also dairy products of ancient usage. Pots of cheese were found in the Second Dynasty tomb at Saqqara (Egypt), while other finds indicate that this important storage food was also eaten in Mesopotamia. Finds of the remains of cheese from the late Bronze Age on the island of Therasia in Greece show how cheese-making developed early in that country. The Brothwells even give us a recipe of Homer's, consisting of: "barley-meal, honey, Pramnian wine and grated goat's milk cheese," adding that "by Roman times, cheese satisfied both the appetite of the peasant and the refined tastes of the gourmet. . . ."

And so, we see that milk and dairy products are ancient foods, appreciated greatly in varying cultures. We must not forget this the next time a dairy prohibitionist admonishes our proclivity for one of man's most important foods. Better we turn the argument to eliminating contaminants from our feedlots than debate the obvious.

Other dietary prejudices, in their turn, have found their way into current dietary therapeutics. Exploiting the widespread popular disapproval of the excesses of Western civilization in the face of so much hunger in the world, the New Age practitioner concentrates her assault on meat-eating and the consumption of alcohol.

*Meat and Wine Defended*

These prohibitions were gladly accepted by many overfed, once indulgent Americans. By giving up these "evils" of the ignorant, neophytes believed they were on the road to a higher state of civilization if not consciousness. Yet meat and alcohol have fueled several dominant cultural groups, not just in warfare, but in the building of significant civilizations. For example, according to Omar V. Garrison, "in early Vedic times, the virile Indo-Aryans who were responsible for Indian civilization at its highest level, were meat eaters and wine drinkers." This is *not* to argue that excessive meat-eating or wine-drinking is healthful. It is a matter of proportion and relative purity. We must seek balance in our aim to restructure health patterns, not by rushing into untried dietary theories, many of which come to us unchallenged. Our new faith and devotion to a better state of health may prosper more from a cleaner food supply and ethnic dietetics than mere dietary prohibitions.

*Inordinate Food Concerns Selfish*

Food needs are extremely individual once we learn to separate our true food needs from what we have learned or been conditioned to believe our needs are. Besides, health and well-being may lie outside a well-balanced meal! This overconcern with food is an expression of wealth. Countless millions make do on mere gruel with occasional highly proteinaceous additions and with lower indices of the diseases of affluence.

Prisoners confined to "strict regime labor camps" in the Soviet Union, working nine hours daily at hard labor, are maintained on a starvation diet of just 1,200 calories, where a minimum of 2,800 calories are required. The point is, while such a starvation regimen is horrendous for the health of the prisoners, they can survive. We would all do better by eating less, concentrating on legislation aimed at purifying our foods, and paying less attention to our every quirk.

Holistic healers and their medical cousins would do well to reevaluate their concepts. Many vitamins and minerals are the waste products of industrial processes! What is advised as healthful may be derived from a sea of waste. Millions are now consuming pellets, like rodents in cages, actually going a step beyond fast foods within a movement claiming closer origins to the earth.

In place of X rays we see the hair analysis; instead of ordering often needless blood tests, the holistic practitioner often orders serum levels of every known vitamin and mineral. For every mode of traditional medicine an alternative mode has been substituted, all within the norms of the medical model. To rescue "alternative" healing, the medical model must be bypassed, and alternative healthways redirected to basics.

Giving much dietary advice myself, I am among the rank and file of this new health movement. The purpose of this brief excursion in criticism is to redirect the good ship *Health* back to its relatively inexpensive origins. Just as Lynceus, pilot-seer of the Argonauts, was needed to sight dangers, we too must learn to see the dangerous trends in alternative medicine, and steer around the shoals of danger.

*Holistic Health Must Be Redirected*

# POSTSCRIPT: ABOARD A SHIP TO PANAMA

I completed the manuscript for this book aboard a passenger freighter bound for Panama. Having driven myself (and everybody around me) half mad with conflicting dietary approaches for the nearly ten years since my father's early death, I wanted some solitude to gain perspective on what has become a study of humanity, not just diet. Food, man and culture, politics, science and the arts are all intimately interrelated. To study only diets without *also* looking at the other elements in the lives of people and then attempt to draw a useful set of coordinates for my clients, can be misleading and dangerous.

About three days south of Los Angeles I drifted into an easy conversation with a well-tanned passenger who seemed very kindly and devoted to his wheelchair-ridden wife. As the tip of Baja disappeared off the port side I realized the groundwork of my ethnic dietary approach was being threatened *again!* This man of seventy-seven, who looked to be about fifty-five, I learned, ate the most atrocious diet I ever personally encountered, and yet he seemed to be in cheerful good health!

"You can count the foods I eat on the palm of your hand," he told me, smiling. "Bread, meat, potatoes, and pastry—it's all I live on—and nobody ever takes me for within fifteen years of my age," the tanned seventy-seven-year-old continued, happy with his new listener. "I don't eat a vegetable every ten years . . . never a piece of fish or seafood in my life . . . salami sandwiches for the last thirty years. I *never* eat food I've never tasted. True, I had gout, but that's why I take these cruises. . . . I feel good in the sun. I used to have three gout attacks a week, thirty years ago. I was on crutches. But since I started worshiping the sun I take much less gout medicine."

How could I continue to suggest that people learn about "diets around the world" and borrow those elements which suited them and which were wisely adaptive to human health? Here was a perfect example of the opposite! A man who ate meat and potatoes all of his life, never a vegetable, no dairy, and he abhorred vitamin supplements as though they were heroin tablets!

Staring at the rolling cobalt waves, I was tempted to quietly drop the 100,000 or so words—the product of three years—and all of my nutrition reference works over the side. "The hell with this entire field," I thought, "it's as unpredictable as mankind! I'll just concentrate on folk medicine, which is far more concrete, and eat as I like, taking my chances."

A bit more reflection saved me from actualizing this impulse. "Another nutritional rogue," I realized, "is who he is. I've found another anomaly blessed with good protoplasm who can violate all apparently sound dietary laws with relative impunity." Finding myself on safer ground, my shaken confidence returned and with it my reasoning faculty. "Why, this man is actually a perfect example of someone who could be particularly well advised with specific nutritional counseling," I reasoned. "True, he is seventy-seven and looks fifty-five, but he has suffered from crippling gout for thirty years, directly as a result of his high-purine diet! Perhaps with some proportional shifts, away from uric acid-producing foods, and minor supplementation* this smiling man could live to the age of Moses without further debilitation!"

And so the manuscript was resumed. Whether you are blessed with good or poor protoplasm, you can probably benefit from this reading. The trick is, do not fall under the spell of messianic "nutritionists" who would have you follow *their* brand of dietary salvation, including a bagful of supplements, usually from their own office! Learn who you are ethnically, learn from other ethnic groups, draw on the biochemical wisdom that is *slowly* evolving, and map your own dietary plan. But above all, please enjoy what you eat, never abandoning our last great unregulated pleasure.

---

* Particularly calcium. He told me his attacks were almost eliminated when he sunned himself. Vitamin D, or calciferol, is activated by sunlight.

# BIBLIOGRAPHY

ANDERSON, J. N. 1977. "Tropical Fruits and Biocultural History." Unpublished manuscript.

BARNICOT, N. A. 1969. "Human Nutrition: Evolutionary Perspectives." *The Domestication of Plants and Animals.* P. J. Ucko and G. Dimbleby, editors. Chicago: Aldine Publishing.

BODENHEIMER, F. S. 1951. *Insects As Human Food.* The Hague: Dr. W. Junk, Publishers.

BOGERT, L. J. 1967. "How Prevalent Is Allergy Among United States School Children?" *Clinical Pediatrics 6:*140.

BOGERT, L. J., BRIGGS, G. M., AND CALLOWAY, D. H. 1979. *Nutrition and Physical Fitness.* 10th ed. Philadelphia: Saunders.

BOYLE, R. 1680. *The Sceptical Chymist.* Oxford, England.

BROTHWELL, D., AND SANDISON, A. T. 1967. *Diseases in Antiquity.* Springfield, Ill.: Charles C Thomas, Publishers.

BROTHWELL, D. AND P. 1969. *Food in Antiquity.* London: Thames & Hudson.

CAHILL, G. F. 1978. "Famine Symposium—Physiology of Acute Starvation in Man." *Ecology of Food and Nutrition 6:*221–230.

CAMERON, E., AND PAULING, L. 1979. *Cancer and Vitamin C.* Menlo Park, California: Linus Pauling Institute.

CHANG, K. C. (ed.). 1977. *Food in Chinese Culture.* New Haven, Connecticut: Yale University Press.

CHERASKIN, E., RINGSDORF, W. M., AND CLARK, J. W. 1968. *Diet and Disease.* New Canaan, Connecticut: Keats Publishing Company.

CHIU-NAN LAI. 1978. "Chlorophyll: The Active Factor in Wheat Sprout Extract Inhibiting the Metabolic Activation of Carcinogens In Vitro." *Nutrition and Cancer 1*(3).

CLEAVE, T. AND CAMPBELL, G. 1966. *Diabetes, Coronary Thrombosis and the Saccharine Disease.* Wright and Sons, Publishers.

COHEN, A. M. 1961. "Prevalance of Diabetes Among Different Ethnic Jewish Groups in Israel." *Metabolism 10:*50.

COMAR, C. L., AND RUST, J. H. 1973. "Natural Radioactivity in the Biosphere and Foodstuffs." In: NAS.

FARNSWORTH, N. R. 1968. "Folk Medicines: Credible or Incredible?" *Tile & Till 54*(3):58–61.

FREDERICKS, C., AND BAILEY, H. 1965. *Food Facts and Fallacies.* New York: Galahad Books.

FREDERICKS, C., AND GOODMAN, H. 1969. *Low Blood Sugar and You.* New York: Grosset & Dunlap.

FREUD, S. 1939. *Moses and Monotheism.* New York: Knopf.

GARRISON, O.V. 1964. *Tantra: The Yoga of Sex.* New York: Julian Press.

GASTER, T. H. 1955. *Customs and Folkways of Jewish Life.* New York: William Sloane.

GOODHART, R. S., AND SHILS, M. E. 1980. *Modern Nutrition in Health and Disease.* 5th ed. Philadelphia: Lea & Febiger.

GOODMAN, R. M. 1979. *Genetic Disorders Among the Jewish People.* Baltimore and London: Johns Hopkins University Press.

GRUSKIN, B. 1940. "Chlorophyll: Its Therapeutic Place in Acute and Suppurative Disease." *American Journal of Surgery* 49:49–55.

GUGGENHEIM, Y. K. 1979. "Forerunners of the Vitamin Doctrine." *Bulletin of Historical Medical Science* 7:634–643.

HEIZER, R. F. 1978. "Man the Hunter-gatherer; Food Availability vs. Biological Factors." *Progress in Human Nutrition,* S. M. Margen and R. A. Ogar, editors. Westport, Connecticut: AVI.

HIGGINSON, J. 1968. "Distribution of Different Patterns of Cancer." *Israel Journal of Medical Science* 4(3):457–466.

HORROBIN, D. F., ET AL. 1979. "The Nutritional Regulation of T Lymphocyte Function." *Medical Hypotheses* 5:969–985.

JACOBSEN, MICHAEL, AND ANDERSON, JOEL. 1972. *The Chemical Additives in Booze.* Washington, D.C.: Center for Science in the Public Interest.

JAFFÉ, W. G. 1973. "Toxic Proteins and Peptides." In: NAS.

JARVIS, D. C. 1960. *Arthritis and Folk Medicine.* Greenwich, Connecticut: Fawcett Crest.

KAPLAN, L. 1969. "Ethnobotanical and Nutritional Factors in the Domestication of American Beans." *Man and His Foods.* C. E. Smith, Jr., editor. University of Alabama Press.

KAUFMAN, W. 1949. *The Common Form of Joint Dysfunction: Its Incidence and Treatment.* Brattleboro, Vermont: Hildreth.

LEARY, T. 1931. "The Therapeutic Value of Alcohol." *New England Journal of Medicine* 205:231.

LESLIE, C. (ed.) 1977. *Asian Medical Systems.* Berkeley: University of California Press.

LOVENBERG, W. 1973. "Some Vaso- and Psychoactive Substances in Food: Amines, Stimulants, Depressants and Hallucinogens." In: NAS.

LUCIA, S. 1954. *Wine as Food and Medicine.* New York: Blakiston.

MALHOTRA, S. L. 1967. "Serum Lipids, Dietary Factors and Ischemic Heart Disease." *American Journal of Clinical Nutrition* 20:462.

MALHOTRA, S. L. 1967. "Geographical Aspects of Acute Myocardial Infarction in India, with Special Reference to the Pattern of Diet and Eating." *British Heart Journal* 29:777.

MAY, J. M. 1961. *The Ecology of Malnutrition.* 5 vols. New York: Hafner.

MILLER, J. J. 1976. *Nutrition vs. Tooth Decay.* West Chicago, Illinois: Medical Modalities.

MODAN, B. 1974. "Role of Ethnic Background in Cancer Development.* *Israel Journal of Medical Science.*

MORGAN, AGNES FAY. 1957. "Utilization of Calories from Alcohol in Wines and Their Effects on Cholesterol Metabolism." *American Journal of Physiology.* 189:290–296.

MURAI, M., PEN, F., AND MILLER, C. D. 1958. *Some Tropical South Pacific Island Foods.* Honolulu: University of Hawaii Press.

NATIONAL ACADEMY OF SCIENCES. 1973. *Toxicants Occurring Naturally in Foods.* Washington, D.C.*

NOBLE, R. Y., BEER, C. T., AND CUTTS, J. H. 1958. "Role of Chance Observations in Chemotherapy: *Vinca rosea.*" *Annual of the New York Academy of Science 76:*882–894.

OBERLEAS, D. 1973. "Phytates." In: NAS.

OHSAWA, G. *Zen Macrobiotics.* New York: Ohsawa Federation.

OHTSUKA, R., AND SUZUKI, T. 1978. "Zinc, Copper and Mercury in Oriomo Papuans' Hair. *Ecology of Food and Nutrition 6:*243.

OSUNTOKUN, B. O. 1970. "Deafness in Tropical Nutritional Ataxic Neuropathy." *Tropical Geographical Medicine 22:*281.

PAULING, L. 1978. "An Orthomolecular Physician." *Linus Pauling Institute Newsletter 1*(4):1–3.

PORKERT, M. 1976. In: *Asian Medical Systems,* edited by C. Leslie. Berkeley: University of California Press.

POULSON, O. 1949. *Extrinsic Factors in Carcinogenesis.* London: H. K. Lewis.

PYKE, M. 1972. *Man and Food.* London.

QUIN, P. J. 1959. *Food and Feeding Habits of the Pedi.* Johannesburg: Witwatersand University.

ROBSON, J. R. K., AND WADSWORTH, G. R. 1977. "The Health and Nutritional Status of Primitive Populations." *Ecology of Food and Nutrition 6:*187–202.

ROE, D. A. 1976. *Drug-Induced Nutritional Deficiencies.* Westport, Connecticut: AVI Publishing.

ROGERS, L. L. 1957. "Glutamine in the Treatment of Alcoholism." *Quarterly Journal of Studies on Alcohol 18*(4):581.

ROSENFELD, I., AND BEATH, O. 1964. *Selenium: Geobotany, Biochemistry, Toxicity and Nutrition.* New York: Academic Press.

RUDOLPH, C., JR. 1977. "Trace Element Patterning in Degenerative Diseases." *Journal of the International Academy of Preventive Medicine.*

SCHMIDT-NIELSEN, K., et al. 1964. "Diabetes Mellitus in the Sand Rat Induced by Standard Laboratory Diets." *Science 143:*689.

---

* Note that all references to NAS are to this particular publication of the National Academy of Sciences.

SEDGWICK, W. T., TYLER, H. W., AND BIGELOW, R. P. 1939. *A Short History of Science*. New York: Macmillan.

SHAMBERGER, R. J., AND FROST, D. V. C. 1969. "Possible Protective Effect of Selenium Against Human Cancer." *Canadian Medical Association Journal 100:*682.

SHENNAN, D. H., AND BISHOP, O. S. 1974. "Diet and Mortality from Malignant Disease in 32 Countries." *West Indies Medical Journal 13:*44–53.

SHIVE, W., ET AL. 1957. "Glutamine in Treatment of Peptic Ulcer." *Texas State Journal of Medicine 53:*840.

SIMOONS, F. J. 1961. *Eat Not This Flesh*. Madison, Wisconsin: University of Wisconsin Press.

STAGG, G. AND MILLIN, D. 1975. "The Nutritional and Therapeutic Value of Tea—A Review." *Journal of Science Food Agriculture 26:*1439–1459.

WEIJERS, H. A., VAN DE KAMER, J. H., MOSSEL, D. A. A., AND DICKE, W. K. 1960. "Diarrhoea Caused by Deficiency of Sugar Splitting Enzymes." *Lancet 2:*296.

WEINER, M. A. 1976. *Bugs in the Peanut Butter: Dangers in Everyday Food*. Boston: Little, Brown.

WEST, K. M. 1972. "Epidemiologic Evidence in Diabetes." *Nutrition and Diabetes Mellitus*. VI Capri Conference.

WILLIAMS, R. J. 1973. *Nutrition Against Disease*. New York: Bantam.

WINE ADVISORY BOARD. 1967. *Uses of Wine in Medical Practice*. 5th ed. San Francisco: Wine Advisory Board.

WOOT-TSUEN WU LEUNG. 1964. *Some Native Foods in East and Southeast Asia—How Nutritious Are They?* Bethesda, Maryland: National Institutes of Health.

YOSHIDA, O., BROWN, R. R., AND BRYAN, G. T. 1971. "A Possible Role of Urinary Metabolites of Tryptophan in the Heterotropic Recurrence of Bladder Cancer in Man. *American Journal of Clinical Nutrition 24:*848.

YUDKIN, J. 1972. *Sweet and Dangerous*. London: Wyden.

YUTANG, L. 1937. *The Importance of Living*. New York: John Day.

# INDEX

aborigines, Australian, diet of, 14
acetylcholine, 162
acid-base balance, 172–176
  ideal, 174
  in individual foods (table), 174–176
acidosis, 223
acupuncture, 229, 232
adrenaline, 66
aflatoxins, 34, 192
Africa:
  cancer in, 192
  diet in, 31–33
agriculture, efficiency of, 17
alcohol, 113–123
  abstention from, 113–114, 234
  cancer and, 189
  exempt from labeling laws, 119, 120–121
  interaction of drugs and, 115, 157
  mineral waters as substitute for, 111
  nuts consumed with, 117
  see also beer; wine
alcoholism, 65–66
allergies, 146–152
  alcohol and, 118–119, 120
  to amines, 149–150, 151
  defined, 146
  to enzymes, 149, 150
  to gluten, 149, 150–152
  as multifactorial, 147
  symptoms of, 147–148
  tests for, 146–147, 148–149
Alvarez, C. R., 211–212
American Cancer Society, 185
Ames bacteria test, 181

amines, 149–150, 151
amino acids (A.A.'s), 42, 58–59
ancient civilizations:
  diet in, 36–42, 233
  herbal remedies in, 183, 184
  medical profession in, 230–231
  milk products in, 232–234
  mineral waters in, 111–112
  nutritional therapy in, 37, 38–39, 142
  wine in, 114
anorexia nervosa, 115
antacids, 93
antibiotics, in livestock feeds, 135–136
anti-folates, 103
antioxidants, 64
apricots, 196
Aretaeus the Cappadocian, 118
arsenic, 88–89, 90, 101, 191
arteriosclerosis, 117, 154, 168
arthritis, 88, 90, 213
asari poison, 137
asbestos, 107
ascorbic acid, see vitamin C
Asia, diet in, 23–24
atherosclerosis, 21, 26, 64, 153–154, 155, 162
  defined, 153
  see also heart attacks; heart disease
Atiu islanders, diet of, 22–23
Atkins, Dr., 225–226
auto-oxidation, 64

back pain, 213
beans, protein in, 42, 59

Bedouins, diet of, 27, 28
beef:
 fattiness of, 60
 inefficiency in production of, 59–60
beer, 119–123
 additives and preservatives in, 121–122
 allergies and, 120
 history of, 119, 121
 nitrosamines in, 119–120
beriberi, 24, 25, 164
betel nuts, 23
BHA, 64
BHT, 64
"bioelectronic theory of life," 180
biotin, 77
birth control pills, 93–94
Bishop, O. S., 193, 194
blood clots, 100–101
Bolendas, diet of, 32
Book of Knowledge (Maimonides), 39–41
bowel gas, 188–189
Boyle, R., 230
bran, 70–71
breadfruit, 22
breast-feeding, acculturation and, 33
Bureau of Alcohol, Tobacco, and Firearms, 119
Bushmen, diet of, 14
butter, 25, 26, 64
buttermilk, 25, 67

cadmium, 88, 90, 101, 213
Cahill, G. F., 160, 223
calcium, 55, 84, 213
 metabolism and absorption of, 26, 70, 73
 -phosphorus ratio, 61–62, 101, 221–222
 as protective nutrient, 22, 63
 sources of, 22, 23, 24, 50, 67, 84
 toxicity of, 88
calories, defined, 56
Cameron, Ewan, 168, 178–179
cancer, 94, 158, 177–196
 bowel gas and, 188–189
 caloric intake and, 194
 in children, 16
 chlorophyll and, 180–181
 cultural differences and, 34–35, 188

cancer—Continued
 electron transfers and, 180–181
 environmental factors in, 106
 ethnic factors in, 194–195
 fat intake and, 62, 187, 188, 194
 fiber intake and, 16, 69, 70, 154
 folic acid and, 103, 184
 food additives and, 16, 130–131, 133, 189–191
 herbal remedies against, 183–185
 immune system and, 178–179, 181–183
 laetrile and, 195–196
 nutrition in causation of, 185–188, 189–195
 occupational hazards and, 186
 in primitive peoples, 15–16
 regional variations in incidence of, 188, 190
 "selective factor" hypothesis and, 192–193
 selenium and, 89, 90
 vitamin C and, 34, 168, 177–180, 182, 191
 see also carcinogens
carbohydrates, 55, 56, 65–71
 classes of, 65
 fat formation and, 63
 see also fiber; starch; sugars
carcinogens, 89, 135
 cooking methods and, 187, 191
 in drinking water, 106
 see also cancer
cardiovascular disease, see heart disease
carotenoid pigments, 132, 134
cassava, 196
Cathcart, William, III, 165–168
"celebration foods," 19–20
cellulose, 65, 70
Central America, ancient, diet in, 42
Challem, Jack, 212–214
champagnes, 116
Chang, K. C., 37–38
channa, 25
chaparral, 183
charcoal broiling, 187
Chatterjee, Pundit, 233
Chemical Additives in Booze, The (Jacobsen), 120–121

chemical bonds, 57
chemicalized foods, 7, 124–134
    amorality of scientists and physicians
        and, 126
    artificial coloring in, 130–134, 163
    disease and suicide caused by, 126
    gradual weaning from, 125
    history of, 127
    industries in promotion of, 124–125
    man not adapted for, 125
    national malnutrition as result of, 125–
        126
    nutrients removed from, 127
    testing of additives in, 127, 128–130,
        191
chemotherapy, 178–179
China, diet in, 24, 34, 38, 62
    in antiquity, 37–38, 232
chitin, 50
Chiu-Nan Lai, 180–181
chlorine, 105, 107
chlorophyll, 57
    cancer and, 180–181, 183
cholesterol, energy and, 63
cholesterol levels, 101, 117, 168
    fiber intake and, 69, 70
    heart disease and, 63–64, 154, 155–156
    hypertension and, 22–23
    in primitive peoples, 15
    protein intake and, 61
choline, 22, 77, 101, 162
chromium, 84, 88, 161–162
chromosomes, 89
clay, as mineral supplement, 50
climate, diet responsive to, 40
cobalt sulfate, 121, 122
coconuts, fat content of, 20–21
Code of Manu, 138
Cohen, A. M., 30
colds, 166, 167, 168, 177
colors, food, see food colors, artificial
combinations of foods, 42, 50, 199–200
computerized dietary analyses, 217–222
Congo:
    diet in, 31–32
    fermented beverages in, 32
constipation, 41, 69, 88, 154

contamination of food, 124–134
    by processing and preservatives, 125–
        134
    by rodents and insects, 125
    see also chemicalized foods
Coppen, Alec, 158
copper, 84
    depression and, 45
    in oysters, 44–45
Coquilles St.-Jacques, 50
Cox, Winifred, 172–174
culture:
    cancer and, 34–35
    food and, 8, 55, 204, 209
cyclamates, 191

Davis, Adelle, 103–104
Delaney Amendment, 131
depression, 157–158
    nutrients and, 45, 94
DeVita, Vincent, 178
dextrins, 65
diabetes, 31, 162, 213, 220
    dietary changes and, 30–31
    fructose vs. sucrose in, 66
    refined carbohydrates and, 30–31
    wine and, 114–115, 118
diarrhea:
    infant, 33
    vitamin C and, 166, 167
diet books, 225
dieticians, 201–202
disaccharides, 65
disease:
    as blocked energy flow, 55
    see also medical nutrition; specific
        diseases
Drug Enforcement Administration codes,
    92
Drug-Induced Nutritional Deficiencies
    (Roe), 94
drugs:
    interactions of alcohol and, 115, 157
    interactions of nutrients and, 93–94, 95–
        99, 150
    malnutrition induced by, 100
    psychotherapeutic, 157, 162, 164
    smoking and action of, 100

drugs—*Continued*
  synthetic, natural resistance lowered by,
    141

eczema, 146–147
Egypt, ancient:
  diet in, 233
  herbal remedies in, 183, 184
elimination diets, 147, 148, 163
Emerson, Ralph Waldo, 125
energy, 55–57
  in chemical bonds, 57
  cholesterol and, 63
  conversion of, 57
  disease and flow of, 55
  as heat, 56
  life and, 55, 56
  sun as source of, 57
  "sweet tooth" as demand for, 67
Environmental Protection Agency,
    106
enzymes, 58, 107
  as food allergens, 149, 150
epidemics:
  as Divine retribution, 231
  water impurities and, 105
Eskimos, diet of, 15, 30, 50, 61
ethnic diets, 9, 11–12, 18–45
  benefits of, 33–34
  cancer and, 34–35
  "celebration foods" in, 19–20
  complementation in, 42, 50
  from distant past, 36–45
  food taboos in, 32, 43–45
  genetic and cultural differences reflected
    in, 19
  overeating proscribed in, 39, 41
  random borrowing from, 42–43
  reevaluation of, 38
  samples of, 20–33
  seasonality in, 40, 41
  stability of ethnic groups and, 18, 19
  time required for evolution of, 42
  in treatment of illness, 37, 38–39
  universal principles of, 39–41
excretions, 39, 41, 69, 90
  *see also* constipation; diarrhea

exercise:
  after meals, 39–40
  before meals, 39

Fadiman, Clifton, 18
fasting, 222–224
  suggested regimen for, 223–224
  total, 223
fatigue, 213
fats (lipids), 21–22, 55, 56, 60–61, 62–64
  in animal vs. plant proteins, 60–61
  cancer and, 62, 187, 188, 194
  carbohydrates and formation of, 63
  classes of, 62–63
  defined, 62
  heart disease and, 20–23, 25–26, 63, 154,
    155–156, 188, 227
  hydrogenation of, 64
  polyunsaturated vs. monounsaturated,
    63
  saturated vs. unsaturated, 63
fava beans, toxicity of, 28–29
Federal Trade Commission, 88
Feingold, Ben, 163
fertilizers, 89, 90
fiber, 69–71
  bowel movements and, 69, 154
  cancer and, 16, 69, 70, 154
  defined, 69, 70
  sources of, 70, 71
fish:
  mercury in, 40, 209
  *see also* shellfish
fluoridation of water, 107
folic acid, 78, 101, 103, 184
Food and Cosmetic Act (1953), 127, 128–
    129
Food and Drug Administration, 53, 88, 119,
    128–129, 208
food colors, artificial, 130–134
  attractiveness and, 132–133
  cancer and, 130–131, 133
  coal-tar, 131
  damage concealed by, 132
  government certification of, 131–132, 133–
    134
  history of, 131, 132

food colors, artificial—*Continued*
  hyperactivity and, 163
  natural vs. synthetic, 131, 132, 134
*Food in Antiquity* (Brothwell and
    Brothwell), 233
*Food in Chinese Culture* (Chang), 37–38
Ford, Ford Maddox, 18
Freud, Sigmund, 136
fructose, 65–66

galactans, 65
galactose, 65, 66
Galileo, 3
Garrison, Omar V., 233, 234
*Genetic Disorders Among the Jewish People*
    (Goodman), 30
genetics, cancer and, 194–195
germanium, 88
Ghana, diet in, 32
ghee, 25, 26
glucagon, 162
glucose, 65, 66, 68, 69
glucose-6-phosphate dehydrogenase
    (G6PD), 29–30
glucose tolerance factor, 161–162, 213
glucose tolerance tests, 159, 160, 161
glutathione peroxidase, 90
gluten, 149, 150–152
glycerol, 62, 63
glycogen, 65, 68, 162
Goodman, Richard M., 30
grains:
  refining or milling of, 24, 69, 70
  whole, fiber in, 69, 70
GRAS list ("Generally Regarded as Safe"),
    129–130
Greece, ancient:
  diet in, 36–37, 233
  mineral waters in, 111–112
Gruskin, B., 181

Habbanites, favism among, 28–29
hair analysis, 208–214, 222
  advantages of, 210
  of chest and pubic hair, 210
  disease states and, 213–214
  limitations of, 209–210

hair analysis—*Continued*
  trace metal levels and, 209
  types of, 208, 210–212
hair dyes, 209–210
Harris, Seale, 159
Hawkins, David, 164
hay fever, 146, 168
heart, function of, 152–153
heart attacks (myocardial infarctions), 156
  among beer drinkers, 121
  decrease in deaths from, 154–155
  described, 153
  strict diet after, 153–154
heart disease, 90, 101, 107, 152–156, 220
  alcohol and, 115, 118
  cholesterol level and, 63–64, 154, 155–
    156
  culture and temperament in, 118
  fats and, 20–23, 25–26, 63, 154, 155–156,
    188, 227
  in primitive peoples, 15
  protective nutrients and, 21–22, 23, 26,
    63, 89, 152, 155–156, 162
  salt intake and, 153
  *see also* atherosclerosis; hypertension
hemicellulose, 70
hemolytic anemia, 29
hepatitis, infectious, 167–168, 177
herbal remedies, 50, 183–185
Hippocrates, 126
Hippocratic Oath, 126
histamine, 150
Hitler, Adolf, 3
Hodgkin's disease, 185
holistic health, 228, 229–235
  Maimonides as precursor of, 39
  meat and alcohol restricted in, 234
  medical practices in, 235
  milk products restricted in, 232–234
  reevaluation needed in, 234–235
  supplements promoted in, 92
Homer, 111, 233
honey, 41, 65, 67, 68
Hopi Indians, mineral deficiencies among,
    50
hormones, in livestock feeds, 135–136
Horrobin, D. F., 181–182, 227

hospital diets, 144–145
    malnutrition as result of, 144–145
    natural foods needed in, 145
hot foods, cancer and, 34–35
Hunter, J. D., 22–23
hunters and gatherers, see primitive
    populations
Hunzas, cancer among, 196
Huxley, Aldous, 142
Huxley, Thomas Henry, 177
hydrogenation, 64
hyperactivity in children, 162–163
hypercalcemia, 88
hypertension, 90, 117, 213
    cholesterol levels and, 22–23
    modernization and, 23
    in primitive peoples, 15
    see also heart disease
hypochlorite, 105
hypoglycemia, 159–161
    controversy over, 159, 160
    defined, 159
    fasting and, 223
    symptoms of, 159–160, 161
    therapeutic diets for, 160, 161

ICP (inductively coupled argon plasma),
    211–212
imipramine, 100, 158
immune system, 146–147, 189
    chemotherapy and, 178–179
    nutrients needed in, 182–183
    T-lymphocyte defects in, 181–182
immunoglobulins, 147
Importance of Living, The (Lin Yutang),
    37
India:
    diet in, 24–26, 227, 232–233
    fasting in, 222
    heart disease in, 26, 227
influenza, 167
inositol, 78
insomnia, 157
Institute of Food Technology, 129
insulin, 66, 114, 118, 159, 160, 161, 162
intestinal bacteria, 15, 26, 67
inversion, 65
iodine, 85

Iran:
    cancer in, 34, 191–192
    diet in, 26, 191–192
Iraq, mercury levels in, 208–209
iron, 50, 70, 85, 94, 101, 116, 191
Isaiah, 232–233
Israel, diet in, 28–31

Japan, cancer in, 34–35
Jenner, Edward, 125
Jewish dietary laws, see "kosher" food laws
juniper berries, 184

Kelts, Drew, 172–174
ketosis, 223
khoa, 25
kidney (organ), 153
kidney stones, 168
kilocalories (kcal), 56
Klenner, Fred, 166
"kosher" food laws (Jewish dietary laws),
    135–138
    foods prohibited by, 44–45, 136–138, 231
    reinterpretation of, 136, 138
"kosher" foods:
    additives in, 135
    baked products, 136
    beef, 135–136
Kuba, diet of, 31

laban, 27
lactase, 66–67
lactic acid, 66, 67
lactose, 65, 66–67
laetrile, 195–196
Lao Tzu, 127
Larrick, George P., 130
laxatives, 40, 112
lead, 88, 101, 128
lecithin, 63
Lele, 31–32
leukemia, 145, 183, 185
linoleic acid, 62, 63, 227
Lin Yutang, 37, 141
lipids, see fats
lipoproteins, 64
lithium, 83–88, 182
liver (organ), 65, 68, 89, 113

livestock feeds, hormones and antibiotics in, 135–136
locusts, 27
Longevity Institute, 226
Lovenberg, W., 150
lysine, 42, 59

macronutrients, 53, 57–71
  defined, 55
  as polymers, 58
  see also carbohydrates; fats; proteins
magnesium, 22, 63, 85, 88, 117, 213
Maimonides, 39–41, 136, 216
malai, 25
maleic hydrazide, 187–188
Malhotra, S. L., 26, 227
manganese, 86, 88, 89, 213
manic-depressive disorders, 83–88
manioc, 32–33
MAO inhibitors, 150
maraschino cherries, 130–131
margarine, 64
mast, 26
Maurois, André, 112
May, Jacques M., 33
Mayans, agriculture of, 17
Mayer, Jean, 121
Mayo Clinic, 177–179
medical nutrition, 141–176
  acid-base balance in, 172–176
  in ancient civilizations, 37, 38–39, 142
  for food allergies, 146–152
  for heart disease, 152–156
  history of, 143–144
  hospital diets and, 144–145
  limitations of, 168–169
  medical model for, 143–144
  for mental disorders, 156–165
  no absolutes in, 142–143
  patient vs. illness treated in, 141–142
  for selected disorders (table), 170–171
  for viral diseases, 165–168
menstruation, copper levels and, 45
mental disorders:
  depression, 45, 94, 157–158
  food in treatment of, 156–165
  hyperactivity, 162–163
  hypoglycemia, 159–161

mental disorders—Continued
  insomnia, 157
  schizophrenia, 163–165
  stress and, 163–164
  vitamin supplements in treatment of, 164–165
mercury, 88, 90, 208–209
  in fish, 40, 209
methionine, 59, 63
methylmalonic acidemia, 172–174
Mexico, ancient, diet in, 42
micronutrients:
  defined, 55
  see also minerals; RDAs; vitamins
milk products, 232–234
  in China, 38, 232
  fermented, lactose intolerance and, 67
  in India, 25, 26, 232–233
  intestinal flora and, 26, 67
  in Iran, 26
  in Saudi Arabia, 27
milorganite, 90
minerals, 55, 72, 83–91
  in drinking water, 106–107
  hair analysis and, 212–214
  oversupplementation of, 83–89
  sources and functions of (table), 84–87
  as supplements, 83–91, 102
  as toxins, 88–89, 91
  see also RDAs; supplements; specific minerals
mineral waters, see spring waters
Mitiaro islanders, heart disease among, 22–23
Modan, Baruch, 194–195
Moertel, Charles G., 178–179
molasses, 67, 68
molybdenum, 88, 89
mononucleosis, 166, 167, 177
monosaccharides, 65
Mozambique, cancer in, 34, 192
muscatel, 116
muscular dystrophy, 89
mussels, toxins in, 137
myocardial infarctions, see heart attacks

National Academy of Sciences, 4, 25, 51, 107

National Cancer Institute, 177, 178, 183, 185
New Jersey, cancer in, 106
niacin, 24, 79, 101, 164
nicotinic acid, 164
Nigeria, diet in, 32–33
nitrites, 135
nitrosamines, 119–120, 191
Noble, R. Y., 184
nutrients:
  defined, 54–55
  interactions of, 93, 101
  interactions of drugs and, 93–94, 95–99,
    150
  see also macronutrients; micronutrients
Nutrition Against Disease (Williams), 21, 23
nutritional therapy, see medical nutrition
nutritionists, 199–214
  choosing of, 199–203
  computerized dietary analyses by, 217–
    222
  dietitians vs., 201–202
  hair analyzed by, 208–214, 222
  sample data forms used by, 203–208
Nyhan, William, 172–174

obesity, 14, 30
Oceania, diet in, 20–23
Ohtsuka, R., 209
orthomolecular medicine, 164–165
osteoarthritis, 90
osteoporosis, 61, 223
over-eating, 39, 41, 216
oysters:
  copper in, 44–45
  toxins in, 137
ozone, 105

PABA (para aminobenzoic acid), 80
pancreas, 161
pandanus, 22
pantothenic acid, 79
Papua New Guinea, diet in, 14–15, 209
Parkinsonism, 117
Pauling, Linus, 72–83, 164, 165–168, 177–179,
  191
pectins, 65
pellagra, 164
periwinkle, 183, 184–185

Pfeiffer, Carl, 45, 72
pH, see acid-base balance
phenothiazine, 164
Phillips, Dr., 192–193
phospholipids, 62–63, 64
phosphorus, 86
  -calcium ratio, 61–62, 101, 221–222
  in meat, 61–62
phytates, 50, 70, 71
pickling, of vegetables, 24
placebo effect, 148, 165, 169, 200
plant ash, 50
plant medicines, 50, 183–185
Plato, 36–37
Pliny, 111, 132, 233
pneumonia, viral, 166, 177
Polo, Marco, 89
polymers, 58
polysaccharides, 65
pork, taboos on, 44
porotic hyperostosis, 50
port, 116
potassium, 86–87, 117, 153, 213
  protein deficiencies and, 15
Poulson, O., 194
pregnancy, wine prohibited during, 115
primitive populations, contemporary, 13–
  17
  acculturation of, 14, 16
  agriculture practiced by, 13, 17
  dietary changes in, 14
  diseases in, 14, 15–16
  energy balance in, 16–17
  as hunters and gatherers, 13–17
  life expectancy in, 15
Pritikin, Nathan, 225–226
"Pritikin Diet," 226–227
prostaglandin (PG) E$_1$, 182
proteins, 55, 56, 58–62
  in animals vs. plants, 59–61, 62
  deficiencies of, in primitive populations,
    15
  efficiency in production of, 59–60
  fat associated with, 60–61
  needs for, 61
  toxicity of, 61
Puckett, Charles, 213
Pure Food and Drugs Act (1906), 131

Pygmies, diet of, 32
pyridoxine, *see* vitamin B$_6$

rabadi, 25
race, lactose intolerance and, 67
radioactivity:
    in drinking water, 109–111
    in ethnic medicine, 111
Rarotongan islanders, diet of, 22–23
raw (uncooked) foods, 28
RDAs (Recommended Dietary
    Allowances), 51–53, 72–73, 204–205
    focus of, 53
    history of, 51–52
    inadequacies of, 52–53
    meaning of, 52
    misuse of, 52
Red Dye #2, 131, 133
Red Dye #4, 130–131
red tide, 137
religion:
    eating habits and, 43–45, 138, 186–187
    fasting and, 222
    wine as symbol in, 114
    *see also* "kosher" food laws; "kosher"
        foods
*Republic* (Plato), 36–37
rheumatoid arthritis, 88, 90, 213
riboflavin (vitamin B$_2$), 34, 75, 101
rice:
    milled, 24
    parboiled, 24–25
rice bran, 24
Robinson, Arthur, 72–83
Robson, J. R. K., 14, 15, 16
Rodale, J. I., 135
Roe, Daphne, 94
Rome, ancient, mineral waters in, 111–112
Rosenthal, Benjamin, 120–121
Rudolph, Charles, Jr., 213
rumen, 60
Russell, Bill, 213

saliva, 69
salt, restricted intake of, 153
Saudi Arabia, diet in, 27–28
SAXAS (scanning automated x-ray
    analysis spectrometer), 208, 210–211

saxitoxin, 137
*Sceptical Chymist, The* (Boyle), 230
schizophrenia, 163–165
    vitamin supplements in treatment of,
        164–165
Schmidt-Nielsen, K., 30
seasons, diet responsive to, 40, 41
selenium, 55, 89–91, 209
    functions of, 89, 90–91
    in soils and fertilizers, 89–90
    sources of, 91
    toxicity of, 89, 91
Senate Select Committee on Nutrition and
    Human Needs (McGovern
    Committee), 53
Senegal, diet in, 31
serotonin, 157–158, 162
Seventh-Day Adventists, cancer among, 34,
    187, 192–193
sewage, 90, 105
Shamberger, Raymond, 90
shampoos, 209
Shaw, George Bernard, 230
shellfish:
    soft-shell, 50
    taboos on, 44–45, 136–138
    toxins in, 44, 136–138
shells, ground, as supplement, 50
Shennan, D. H., 193, 194
sherry, 116
Shubik, Dr., 189–191
sleep disorders, 157
smoking, 94–101, 189
    ill effects of, 94–101, 113
    interaction of drugs and, 100
    interaction of nutrients and, 100, 101
snacks, meals vs., 13–14
social position, food and, 33
sodium, 87, 117
Solomon, 41
spring (mineral) waters, 107–108
    as medicinal agents, 111–112
    radioactivity in, 109–111
starch, 65, 68–69
strategy for daily dining, 215–217, 228
sucrose, 65–66, 67
sudden infant death, 41

sugars, 65–68
    implicated in diseases, 68
    intolerance to, 66–67
    maple, 67
    sweetness of, 65–66
sulfates, 89, 112
sulfur, 87
sun, as energy source, 57
supplements, 49–104
    amino acids as, 91, 93
    in antiquity, 49–51
    controversy on, 72–73
    excessive doses of, 83–89, 103–104
    formulation recommended for, 101, 102
    glandular extracts as, 91, 93
    promotion of, 91–93
    quality control of, 101–103
    as short-term solution, 141–142
    as substitute for nutrition, 73–83
    see also minerals; RDAs; vitamins
Suzuki, T., 209
"sweet tooth," 67
Szent-Gyorgyi, Albert, 177, 179–180

taboos on foods, 32, 43–44, 136–138, 230–
    231, 232–234
tardive dyskinesia, 162
taro, 22
Tasaday, diet of, 13–14
tea, carcinogens in, 187
tetracyclines, 93
Thailand:
    beriberi in, 24
    cancer in, 192
thiamine, see vitamin B$_1$
titanium, 88
tofu, 60
toxicology, 128–130
    biases in, 129
    governmental responsiveness and, 128–
    129
    inadequacies of techniques in, 128
toxins:
    in drinking water, 106, 107
    individual responses to, 29
    minerals as, 88–89, 91
    in shellfish, 44, 136–138
    vitamins as, 73

tricyclic antidepressants, 157, 158
triglycerides, 62, 154
tryptophan, 42, 101, 157–158, 162
tyramine, 149–150, 151

uranium, 109, 111

vermouth, 116
vinblastine, 185
vincristine, 183, 184–185
viral diseases, vitamin supplements in
    treatment of, 165–168
vitamin A, 34, 73, 74
vitamin B, 74
vitamin B$_1$ (thiamine), 75, 150
    beriberi and, 24, 25, 164
vitamin B$_2$ (riboflavin), 34, 75, 101
vitamin B$_3$, 113, 158
vitamin B$_6$ (pyridoxine), 75–76, 100, 101,
    156, 158, 164
    birth control pills and, 94
    heart disease and, 21, 22, 26, 63, 152, 155–
    156
    national deficiency of, 156
vitamin B$_{12}$ (cobalamin), 55, 76, 100, 101,
    173
vitamin B$_{15}$ (pangamic acid), 80
vitamin C (ascorbic acid), 22, 63, 70, 72,
    80–81, 94, 101
    cancer and, 34, 168, 177–180, 182, 191
    diarrhea and, 166, 167
    normal cell division promoted by, 180
    smoking and, 100, 101
    viral diseases and, 165–168
vitamin D (calciferol), 73, 81, 101
vitamin E (tocopherol), 22, 63, 64, 69, 72,
    81–82, 89, 101, 164
vitamins, 55, 71–83
    deficiencies of, 72, 73, 164
    evolution and need for, 71
    interactions of, 101
    mental disorders and, 164–165
    sources and functions of (table), 74–82
    as supplements, 71–83, 102, 156, 164–168
    toxicity of, 73
    variability in requirements of, 52, 72
    see also RDAs; supplements; specific
        vitamins

water as nutrient, 55, 105–112
  in body composition, 105
  bottled, 107–108
  carcinogens in, 106
  disinfecting agents for, 105, 107
  distilled, 108–109
  filtration systems for, 105–106, 107, 108–109
  fluoridation of, 107
  minerals in, 106–107
  radioactivity in, 109–111
  spring and mineral, 107–108, 109–112
wheat, protein in, 59
wheat juice, 180–181
Williams, Roger, 21–22, 23, 26, 152, 155
  vitamin/mineral formulation of, 101, 102
Wilm's tumor, 185
wine, 114–119
  antibacterial and antiviral activity of, 117–118

wine—*Continued*
  chemical additives in, 118–119
  chemistry of, 115–117
  complaints and contraindication of, 115
  history of, 114
  in hospitals, 118
  medicinal uses of, 114–115, 117–118
  as tranquilizing agent, 114, 115
  types of, 116
World Health Organization, 130

xerophthalmia, 31
XRF (X-ray fluorescence), 208, 210–211

Yemenites, diet of, 28, 30
yogurt, 26, 27, 67
Yudkin, J., 220

zinc, 70, 87, 117, 164, 209, 213
  premenstrual tension and, 45